There's Something Funny About Nutrition

By

Gary Evans

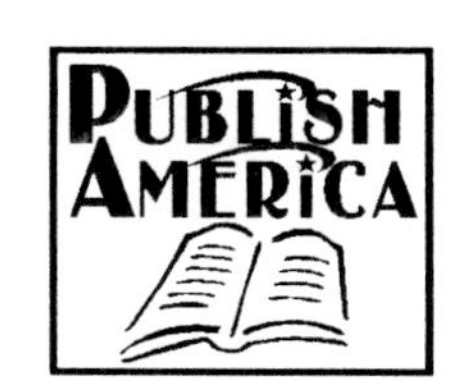

PublishAmerica
Baltimore

First printing

ISBN: 1-59286-264-0
PUBLISHED BY PUBLISHAMERICA BOOK PUBLISHERS
www.publishamerica.com
Baltimore

Printed in the United States of America

Dedication

To Linda—always.

Acknowledgments

I wish to acknowledge the help of all the committees, subcommittees, committee members, authors, organizations and just plain people whose dedication to keeping us healthy has contributed to making nutrition one of the most, if not the most, contentious subjects in science; thereby providing the fodder for this persiflage.

The legally required FDA disclaimer:

"The statements herein have not been evaluated by the Food and Drug Administration. The information contained within this book is not intended to diagnose, treat, cure or prevent disease."

Introduction

IN THE BEGINNING

In the beginning, God populated the earth with broccoli and cauliflower and spinach and green and yellow and red vegetables of all kinds, so Man and Woman would live long and healthy lives.

Then, using God's great gifts, Satan created Ben & Jerry's and Krispy Creme. And Satan said, "You want chocolate with that?" And Man said "Yea." And Woman said, "And another one with sugar sprinkles." And they gained ten pounds.

And God created the healthful yogurt that Woman might keep the figure that man found so fair. And Satan brought forth white flour from the wheat and sugar from the cane, and combined them. And Woman went from size two to size six.

God said, "Try my fresh green salad." And Satan presented Thousand-Island Dressing and garlic toast on the side. And Man and Woman unfastened their belts following the repast.

God then said, "I have sent you heart healthy vegetables and olive oil in which to cook them." And Satan brought forth deep fried fish and chicken-fried steak so big it needed its own platter. And Man gained more weight and his cholesterol went through the roof.

God then brought running shoes so that his children might lose those extra pounds. And Satan gave cable TV with a remote control so Man would not have to toil changing the channels. And Man and Woman laughed and cried before the flickering light, and gained pounds.

Then God brought forth the potato, naturally low in fat and brimming with nutrition. And Satan peeled off the healthful skin and sliced the starchy center into chips and deep fried them. And Man gained pounds.

God then gave lean beef so that Man might consume fewer calories and still satisfy his appetite. And Satan created McDonald's and its 99-cent double cheeseburger. Then said, "You want fries with that?" and Man replied, "Yea! And Super Size 'em." And Satan said, "It's a good thing." And Man went into cardiac arrest. God sighed and created quadruple bypass surgery. And Satan created HMOs.

I was originally going to title this book "Food Flummery" but was worried prospective buyers might have to steal a dictionary from the bookstore to determine what the title meant. For your edification, flummery is "oatmeal or flour boiled with water until thick." I'm serious. That's actually the first of four meanings. The fourth definition and the one I considered using is "complete nonsense." No, the fourth definition isn't complete nonsense, it's, as I stated, "complete nonsense."

There are over four thousand books about nutrition cluttering the shelves of bookstores and libraries. Each one is scholarly, sophisticated, enlightening, educational, drab, tedious and boring. Many (way too many) of these books were written by journalists who write or have written columns about food and nutrition. These people have never been involved with a clinical study but they are skilled at misinterpreting another author's misinterpretation of another author's misinterpretation of the original scientist's results. And they eat.

Many of the authors are also physicians who, despite their lack of training in nutrition, have decided they know more about nutrients than anybody else. And they eat and would rather cure your ailments with their particular vitamin/mineral formulation than put up with the hassles of an HMO. Celebrities who have suddenly taken an interest in our health and well being also write quite a few of the books. Professionals who actually majored in some area of nutritional science, paid attention in class and earned a degree write some of the books.

Regardless of whether they're untrained journalists, physicians, legitimate or illegitimate nutritional scientists, each considers himself a thaumaturge possessing afflatus. No, that's not an intestinal disorder resulting in gas leakage. Using soporific prose that requires a caffeine catheter to wade through, every author extols the virtues of her/his new improved health plan that will cure everything from boils and bunions to butt fungus (Four Days to Better Health; Three Days to Better Health; 2 1/2 Days to Lithe Living; Two Hours to Lissome Limbs [this is a book about liposuction]; Soy Joys; Eat This Book, The Cover Is Made Of Soy).

After retiring a few years ago, I completed a couple of non-fiction books about nutrition topics and then wrote a fictional novel in which vitamin C is the main character (I'm serious). Following completion of the novel, I became restless and wanted to write another book. Because I live in Nevada, writing helps keep me out of the casinos and brothels. I pondered and pouted because all the good stuff had been taken and wondered what I could do to create a unique book about nutrition. Novels are more fun but non-fiction sells better, unless you are John Grisham or Michael Crichton, who, by the way, has successfully written both.

I considered a book in which I would dredge up all the hackneyed topics, write about them in my own style and then throw in a whole bunch of stuff about little known nutrients like lithium (it keeps you mellow, man, and is found in fruits and vegetables and pharmacies) and germanium. Yes, germanium. It hasn't been voted in as an essential nutrient for humans or animals but a lot of studies have shown that it's needed for a lot of things.

While contemplating my navel and eating an orange, it occurred to me nutrition is undoubtedly one of the most controversial subjects known to man. Paraphrasing George Bernard Shaw, if all nutritional scientists were laid end to end, they still wouldn't reach a conclusion. According to Mark Twain "a scientist will never show any kindness for a theory which he didn't start himself." This is certainly true in the nutritional sciences where differing opinions abound regarding how we should get our nutrients, how much we need and whether or not we are getting enough—to name a few.

With all this rancor—rancor is the pus of reason—I decided it was time somebody said, "Hey, lighten up. Have some pie and ice cream." Stressed is desserts spelled backward. So I chucked the germanium idea and decided to annoy nutrition professionals with a persiflage.

This book is divided into three sections. Does that make it a trilogy? "On Becoming An Ist" is a collection of chapters about becoming an Ist. The second section, "Being An Ist," tells you what Ists do. The third section is the appurtenance, consisting of the Glossary and Appendix. There are three appendixes. Or is it appendices? If the plural of ox is oxen why isn't the plural of box boxen? One fowl is a goose, but two are called geese; yet the plural of moose should never be meese. You may find a lone mouse or a nest full of mice; yet the plural of house is houses, not hice. If the plural of man is always called men, why shouldn't the plural of pan be called pen? If I spoke of my foot and show you my feet, and I give you a boot, would a pair be called beet? If one is a tooth and a whole set are teeth, why shouldn't the plural of booth be called beeth? One may be that, and three would be those, yet hat in the plural would never be hose, and the plural of cat is cats, not cose. We speak of a brother and also of brethren, but though we say mother, we never say methren.

There were four appendixes/appendices but one had to be removed. After the appendixes/appendices you come to The End, and by then I think you will believe me when I tell you, "There's something funny about nutrition."

Section One:

ON BECOMING AN IST

Things An Ist Must Learn

What Is Nutrition?

Since the main topic of this book is nutrition, let's be sure everybody knows exactly what nutrition is. Nutrition is many things. Webster's big book, the unabridged dictionary, lists five definitions for nutrition. Little wonder the field is embroiled in controversy with an identity crisis like that.

According to one of my sources, the French chemist Antoine Lavoisier is credited as being the founder of the science of nutrition. Because I want the topics discussed in this book to be factual and accurate (well, some of them) I checked on Antoine. He is actually credited with being the "father of chemistry." (I have no information regarding the mother). Biochemistry is a branch of chemistry and nutrition science is a branch of biochemistry, therefore Lavoisier is more than likely nutrition's great-grandfather. (Again, no information about the grandmother).

Lavoisier never discovered any elements or improved any laboratory procedures. He did, however, interpret (some have called it stealing) other scientists' experiments. Lavoisier named 33 different elements including oxygen and hydrogen. He explained how oxygen burns and invented Plaster of Paris. Lavoisier was a theorist; he told people sodium and potassium would soon be discovered—five years later they were. He also did some experiments that led to his writing what chemists call "the law of conservation of mass." The law had to be revised, though, because a guy named Albert Einstein kept breaking it.

When Lavoisier wasn't predicting, stealing, writing laws or fathering, he kept busy earning a living as a tax collector for King Louis XVI. This was not a very popular (or smart) vocation during the French revolution so Lavoisier was among the first to be introduced to Monsieur Guillotine's cutting edge invention.

Before the revolutionists chopped off his head, Lavoisier showed what water was made of. This angered many in France who love the fruit of the vine. It seems word got around that Lavoisier was undermining the production and drinking of wine by claiming that water was made from two kinds of gin, oxy gin and hydro gin.

Ists

Several years ago, I was scheduled to be interviewed via telephone about a discovery I'd made—chromium picolinate—in the field of nutrition. I knew from the pre-interview chatter between the hostess and her radio technician that this was not going to be an easy exchange. The hostess was obviously having a bad day and let the technician know with the use of several expletives.

A few seconds before the interview was to begin, the hostess made a statement and said something about me being a nutritionist. I responded with, "Whatever that is."

"Well, aren't you a biochemist?" she demanded.

"Yes," I replied.

"Then you're a nutritionist," she stated.

"I suppose," I reluctantly agreed.

"Well, my husband is a biochemist," she reported, "and he considers himself a nutritionist."

The interview went downhill from that point. Twice she referred to chromium picolinate as a drug and twice I assured her it wasn't a drug. Following the second denial of chromium picolinate being a drug, the hostess said, "I don't like your attitude" and hung up.

Afterward, I looked up the term and sure enough the rude hostess was right. One of Webster's definitions for nutrition includes the kinds of things done in the biochemistry lab. The same Mr. Webster defines nutritionist (nutrition + ist) as anyone who studies or is an expert in the field of nutrition. The term was coined sometime in the late 1920s, apparently because some expert or someone studying nutrition felt threatened or insecure when asked what their job was. After all, an expert in physics is a physicist, an expert in chemistry is a chemist and in my field we specialists are called biochemists.

But why nutrition + ist? The authorities in physics had to give up an 's,' both the biology and psychology people lost a 'y' and pity the chemistry and biochemistry professionals who had to forgo two letters, 'r' and 'y.' Why, I have wondered for years, didn't the nutrition expert have to give up at least one letter? Is it not true that the study of nutrition requires input from several sciences such as biochemistry, chemistry, physics and biology? I realize nutritioist is a bit awkward but what's wrong with nutritist? Two letters lost and fair is fair. Nutritionist is elitist (elite – e + ist) and I refuse to acknowledge the term.

While I was writing this section, I wondered why people who study medicine are not medicinists. But then I realized most who study medicine first earn a medical degree and then chose a specialty in which they become Ists: pathologist, neurologist, oncologist, cardiologist, gynecologist, etc.

Also, I should mention my personal dislike for the term expert, the reason being "ex," the prefix, refers to former or has been and Mr. Webster tells there are four meanings for "pert"—three current and one obsolete. One definition is boldly forward in speech or behavior; impertinent or saucy. A second says pert is jaunty and stylish; chic; natty. The third of the currents describes pert as lively; sprightly or in good health. No need to bother with the obsolete because it isn't used anymore, it's obsolete.

Since an expert was once saucy, stylish or in good health but is no more, I choose not to be referred to as such. This self-chosen preference has caused some questions to arise because now hosts and hostesses introduce me, not as an expert in the field of chromium but, as "the father of chromium picolinate." I have no idea how one fathers a nutrient and I'm at a complete loss as to the mother.

Sweet Things

In order to become certified, canonized, legalized, harmonized and lionized Ists, students of the nutritional sciences must learn about carbohydrates, lipids (a.k.a. fats, a.k.a. lipids), proteins, vitamins and minerals. Let's begin with a little trivia about carbohydrates, which are made up of carbon, hydrogen and oxygen. Sometime in the late 1860s, a group of chemists was gathered around a table trying to come up with a name for the plentiful substance they had discovered in plants and animals. They consulted their Greek and Latin dictionaries, tried to think of some dignified scientist they could honor but there was no agreement. During these deliberations, one of the scientists was doodling on a scrap of paper. Suddenly he jumped up, rushed to the chalkboard and wrote $C H_2O$, which showed the atomic makeup of these substances. Pointing to the 'C' he said, "Carbo." Pointing to the H_2O he stated, "Hydrate." Raising his hands in jubilation he shouted, "We'll name the substance carbohydrate!"

The others gathered around the table wishing they had thought of that and responded with, "Well, duh."

All substances that are carbohydrates have names that end with 'ose,' except for starch, glycogen, chitin, hyaluronic acid, chondroitin sulfate, inulin, heparin and a whole bunch of others.

The textbooks tell us there are simple carbohydrates and complex carbohydrates. Don't believe it; they're all complex. Consider for example the so-called "simple sugars." There are trioses, tetroses, pentoses, hexoses, heptoses, aldoses, and ketoses. There are fourteen different simple sugars with names like arabinose (found in dates grown on an oasis), galactose (found in meteorites) and mannose (soon to be renamed "personose").

Moving up a step in the complexity of carbohydrates we have the disaccharides. Di is Greek for two and saccharide is Greek for sugar, so there you have it. Some of the more important disaccharides are sucrose (found in healthy vegetables like sugar cane and sugar beets), lactose (found in milk), maltose (found in milk shakes) and trehalose (the major sugar of insect hemolymph).

After the disaccharides come the polysaccharides, named for the daughter of a scientist who did a lot of work with carbohydrates. Starch (used to make collars stiff) is a polysaccharide. So is glycogen (animal starch but it isn't used to stiffen collars). Cellulose is another polysaccharide found in plants but humans can't digest it. The same is true of chitin, an indigestible polysaccharide found in crustaceans and insect skeletons. Nutrition experts tell us we need "bulk" or fiber in our diets. You can get these by eating whole vegetables and grasshoppers.

Discussions of carbohydrates were once simple but now they are complex. Thirty years ago nutrition scientists and professors, including this author, urged their students and other citizens to get about 60% of their total caloric intake from carbohydrates and most followed this advice. That was until Robert Atkins, Barry Sears and the husband/wife teams of Hellers and Eades persuaded people to eat diets that contain half as much carbohydrate, or better, none at all. The people who promote the low carbohydrate diets believe carbohydrates promote insulin production and high blood insulin levels make you fat. "Cut the carbs and you'll cut the fat," they state.

Who knows, maybe the low-carb people are right, even if for the wrong reasons. According to a report out of Sweden, high carbohydrate foods that have been cooked—potato chips, French fries, biscuits and bread—contain a chemical called acrylamide. Acrylamide is a substance used by research scientists in a procedure known as electrophoresis. Obviously, the body doesn't do this so it's considered dangerous material that causes cancer. The Swedish scientists issued the report long before the study had been reviewed by peers and published in a journal. According to the Swedes, they thought it was important enough to issue a preliminary statement and scare the beejesus out of everybody who has ever eaten cooked carbohydrates. (The last part was not Swedish.)

The media, always willing to embellish disturbing news, especially when it comes to our diets, dutifully announced that starchy foods, cooked at high temperatures, might contain carcinogens. "There's more on French fries than ketchup," the headlines proclaimed. There weren't any acrylamides in meat, poultry or fish but then they're already stuffed full of nitrates and mercury so there isn't room for any more toxic junk. Most of the responsible experts, those outside the media that is, are telling us not to get too excited about the Swedish report; as long as we don't eat French fries and potato chips every day.

The people who oppose consumption of low carbohydrate foods feel the diets drain our systems of calcium—nutrition professionals seldom suggest using supplements—and subject us to dangerous chemicals and microbes found in meat and other high protein foods. These folks apparently don't consider the herbicides and pesticides used in crop production as posing any hazard. Also, the problem of genetically manipulated (GM) foods is overlooked.

Carbohydrates are one of the most controversial topics in nutrition science today. (Enter the Zone; No, stay out of the Zone, you'll get mugged.) While the economy struggles, corporations steal retirement funds from employees, Microsoft doesn't work and people are starving, nutrition experts hotly debate whether or not carbohydrates are unhealthy. There will be more about this later, after our budding young students become certified Ists.

Fats

If you were to pick up a textbook on nutrition science and look for a chapter on fats you wouldn't find one. The chapter you'd be looking for would be titled "Lipids." Lipids are defined as any group of organic compounds that are greasy to the touch, insoluble in water and soluble in alcohol or ether. Lipid comes from the Greek word *lipos*, for fat. Fat has been around for a long time. The term, I mean. Fat is derived from the old English *faetan*, which means to cram, load or adorn. Lipid entered the scientific language sometime in the late 1920s. Some scientist probably whined to the Committee That Names Stuff that he'd been called a fat chemist.

Lipid is a useful term; consider the class of proteins that carry fat through the blood. They're called apolipoproteins. After fat attaches to one of these transporters they're called lipoproteins. Those terms have a much more sophisticated sound than apofatproteins or fat proteins.

The language of lipids is a murky one. Chapters on lipids usually begin with the statement that the correct term for fats is lipids but a few paragraphs later the authors write about fatty acids, not lipidy acids. There are saturated fatty acids (sat. fats), EFAs and PUFAs. When I see the term PUFA I think of the colorful fish I see while snorkeling off the coast of Maui. The omega-3 fatty acids found in female salmon (salmonellas) are PUFAs.

EFAs are the essential fatty acids. These are the big molecules that our body can't make so we must get them from our diet. The

PUFAs are the polyunsaturated fatty acids. These are liquid fats (a.k.a. lipids) found in vegetable oils. As if all these terms aren't enough to short circuit our synapses, we also have cis and trans fatty acids. The body makes the cis variety but the trans fatty acids are produced when manufacturers try to make artificial PUFAs.

Trans fatty acids began appearing in our blood streams way back when the professionals started preaching about the harmful effects of saturated fats. Now, after 50 years of pouring liquid fats down our gullets, we're being told trans fatty acids are more harmful than the saturated variety. More about this later.

Another mind boggler in the lipid lexicon is triglyceride. Tri comes from the Latin *tres* or *tria* or the Greek *treis* or *tria* meaning, you guessed it, three. Glyceride doesn't come from Greek, Latin, German, Danish or any other lingo. It's the biochemical term for glycerol, which is not a lipid (a.k.a. fat) at all; it's an alcohol, but not at all like beer or gin. Glycerol is a small molecule with three chemical hooks on it that grab and hold long chains of fatty acids. Fatty acids are moved through blood and tucked away in your butt, thighs and tummy as triglycerides. When a physician says, "Mrs. Fritinzimmer, you have an inordinately elevated level of serum triglycerides," it's simply the doctor's snooty way of saying, "You have too damn much fat in your blood, Porky."

We also have phospholipids. These are lipids that have a few atoms of phosphorous attached. They're the bricks and mortar that are used to make the walls around cells to keep important chemicals from leaking out and garbage from sneaking in. The most famous phospholipid is lecithin. Years ago, after scientists discovered lecithin in brain cells, several companies started marketing the product as an aid to brain development and memory capacity. A student of mine once informed me he took lecithin supplements before exams. He graduated with honors and is now an executive in a company that manufactures scientific apparatus.

The term lipid really has turned out to be a good addition to scientific jargon. When a group of fat chemists are standing around at a party sipping cocktails and talking shop, phospholipid sounds much more scholarly than phosphofat. Also, people who worry about fat, either in their food on their bodies, are lipophobes not fatophobes.

The fats (a.k.a. lipids, a.k.a. fats) we eat or make inside our bodies are stored in little lipid larders called adipose cells or adipocytes. Adipose is Latin for fat (I told you lipid language is murky). Why the cells are called adipose, I do not know. Lipocytes would work fine but somebody who marched to the sound of a different drummer decided we needed to throw in some Latin and brought in adipose. Most likely a descendant of some Roman emperor, the adipose person probably envisioned a bunch of Greeks crowded into Roman cells.

For years, people who carried around too much adipose tissue (that's a whole bunch of adipose cells gathered together) were called fat. The era of politically correct ushered in a new term for those nutritional overachievers. Nowadays, people are not fat; they are "obese" or if they have way too many adipocytes, they're "morbidly obese." When obese goes out of style, I suggest we call these overweight lipid larders "adipocytically challenged." That should catch on.

And what about cellulite, pronounced SELL-you-leet. You know what sell means; leet is just another word for junk. Some people pronounce it SELL-you-LITE, which has the same connotation, lite meaning little. The term is derived from a greed word meaning swindle. According to several unscrupulous marketers, there are two kinds of fat: regular fat and cellulite. When adipocytes are really thick in some spots, they get attached to the skin and pull it inward. This causes the skin to look lumpy ("serious hail damage" my son calls it). Marketers who want you to join their spa or buy their massagers claim the fat in cellulite must be broken up before it can be "burned up" and eliminated. Cellulite is listed in dictionaries but they'll correctly tell you it isn't a medical term.

The most expensive addition to the world of lipids is olestra. Olestra is a fat that isn't. It has all the qualities of fat but can't be absorbed, so no lard gets into the blood. Scientists at Proctor & Gamble, the folks who are best known for laundry detergents, discovered it at a cost of over $200 million. I'm not positive, but I think olestra comes from a foreign word that means "flim flam." Olestra, because it resembles fat, hooks up with taste proteins that send a message to the brain informing it a meal of fat is being eaten.

Brain cell one, "Wow! That was really tasty."

Brain cell two, "Nothing like fat to satisfy the ol' appetite."

The idea behind olestra was good but a few problems arose during testing. Researchers discovered that fat-soluble vitamins tend to join up with olestra and get carried out of the body. That's certainly not a trivial problem but is miniscule compared to the others that surfaced. Many of the people involved with the study suffered from, in the words of the scientists, "anal leakage." The molecule is big and dense so enzymes can't break it down in the intestines. As a result "the olestra passed through the gastrointestinal tract and actually stained the underwear of test subjects." Despite the humility of stained underwear, the hapless volunteers were still referred to as "subjects." Researchers at P&G were able to reduce the amount of "anal leakage" and underwear staining, but the problem has not been completely eliminated. Bloating, cramping and diarrhea often occur in individuals who eat as little as an ounce of potato chips made with olestra.

Brain cell one, "We're getting some disturbing messages from the large intestine. What's going on down there?"

Brain cell two, "The master has the squirts."

Since Proctor & Gamble is in the detergent business, they should be encouraged to develop a special detergent for stains. For marketing purposes, the product could be placed alongside foods prepared with olestra. Names they might consider include: olestra out, stain out, and, of course, poop out.

While I was word processing this work—before the PC era, authors used pithy prose like "penning this piece"—a reader of *The Washington Post* introduced a new term into the lipid dictionary: flabbergasted, an adjective which means to be appalled over how much weight you have gained.

Here's a parting thought for you etymologists. Many of the words and phrases in our language are contractions or truncations of older words and phrases. The human buttocks are comprised primarily of adipocytes filled with fatty acids. Years ago, people in polite society referred to those with big butts as having "fatty acid filled derrieres." That was cumbersome, especially if you wanted to insult somebody. First the derriere was dropped and the big butts were called simply "fatty acids." The phrase crossed continents, sailed the seas and passed through hundreds of dialects eventually surfacing as "fat ass." Can you imagine trying to insult somebody by calling him or her a lipid ass?

Gas From Food

Carbohydrates and fats, phospholipids being an exception, are used primarily as fuel to operate the body cells. All cells need fuel but muscles use the most. We evolved as a species that stores fuel inside the body. Unused carbohydrates and fats are not excreted, they are stored. When operating muscles—lifting, walking, running, picking your nose, scratching your butt—carbohydrates are used first because they are stored near the muscle machinery that needs them. When muscle activity becomes vigorous, fats are unhooked from the triglycerides and delivered to the working muscles. Healthy people eat, store carbohydrates in the muscle and liver, store fats in adipocytes and then use the stored fuel to work or exercise. Unhealthy people eat, store carbohydrates in the muscle and liver, store fats in adipocytes, eat some more and look for ways to shrink their adipocytes without exercising.

Contrary to what adipocytically challenged people (I'm starting my campaign here) would like to believe, there is no chemical that will destroy stored fat. Imagine if somebody were to discover and market such a substance. After the chemical entered the body and started attacking the fat, what would happen? If the stored fat was simply released, the blood vessels would be clogged; blood flow would soon stop and a lard sculpture would be created. If the fat were solubilized and dissolved in the blood fluid, where would the dissolved material go? The kidneys would have no part of those big fat molecules so the gunk would be sent to the liver (those of you who savor liver should keep in mind it's the body's garbage dump). In the liver, the freed fat would be broken into tiny pieces, a process that would generate enough heat to fry the lazy porker. There is, as the saying goes, "no magic bullet." Those who choose not to operate their muscles to drain their fuel tanks can look forward to a life of waddling around with a stomach, thighs and butt packed with Greek lipids stuffed into Roman cells.

The folks in the nutritional sciences like to talk about carbohydrates and fats in terms of calories. A calorie is...never mind, it's not that important. Suffice it to say, calories tell us how much energy foods can produce. It's a little like knowing how many miles you can drive your car on a gallon of gas. Professionals speak of the fuel we get from food in terms of calories per gram (gram is a metric unit and since Congress has refused to adopt that system I'll not bother with any explanations). Carbohydrates have 4000 calories per gram. Fats, with their special additives, have 9000 calories per gram. This was determined by putting various kinds of food into a small stove with a pot of water on it, setting fire to the food and measuring how warm the water became (don't try this at home).

Calorie talk can be confusing. Humans need about two million four hundred thousand calories a day to operate all the machinery. That's a big number (2,400,000) and looked like an awful lot of food, so some nutritionist (nutrition + ist) decided to make calories less overwhelming by stating that humans require only two thousand four hundred kilocalories (that's much better and not so much food). Kilo comes from a Greek word meaning one thousand. Kilo is most often abbreviated 'k' resulting in 2,400 kcalories or super abbreviated, 2,400 kcal.

Because humans consume so many calories—over half the nation is overweight—another nutritionist decided we should have dietary calories, resulting in big calories and little calories (for worms and other very tiny creatures). A big calorie is 1000 calories or a kcal and is written with a capital 'C'. Thus, one dietary Calorie = 1000 calories.

In the metric system, energy is expressed as joules rather than calories. Thus, in the United States, a soft drink machine dispenses diet soda that has less than one Calorie. In countries where they use the metric system, that same diet drink is a low-joule cola. Dieters in countries that don't have metric phobia refuse a second helping of pie and ice cream by expressing a need to watch their joules.

Personally, I feel we should use kcal exclusively and convince people—especially the nutritional overachievers—that the 'k' stands for killer. Tell our fat nation that killer calories (kcal) eaten and stored with no activity to use them will live up to their name.

A sidebar

Some books and many magazines use sidebars or footnotes to stick in little ditties about a subject discussed in the body of the text. I don't care for either so when I intend to give you some extra related (or unrelated) information, I'll call it a sidebar but I won't put it off to the side where you'll have to shift your eyes to read it. Also, you won't be able to purchase drinks at the sidebar.

As we all know, it takes one calorie to heat one gram of water one degree centigrade. Translated into meaningful terms, this means that if you eat a very cold dessert (generally consisting of water in large part), the natural processes which raise the consumed dessert to body temperature during the digestive cycle literally suck the calories out of the only available source, your body fat. For example, a dessert served and eaten at near 0 degrees C (32.2 degrees F) will, in a short time, be raised to the normal body temperature of 37 degrees C (98.6 degrees F). For each gram of dessert eaten, that process takes approximately 37 calories, as stated above. The average dessert portion is six oz, or 168 grams. Therefore, by operation of thermodynamic law, 6,216 calories (one cal./gm/deg. x 37 deg. x 168 g) are extracted from body fat as the dessert's temperature is normalized. Allowing for the 1,200 latent calories in the dessert, the net calorie loss is approximately 5,000 calories. Obviously, the more cold dessert you eat, the better off you are and the faster you will lose weight, if that is your goal.

This process works equally well when drinking very cold beer in frosted glasses. Each ounce of beer contains 16 latent calories, but extracts 1,036 calories (6,216 cal. per 6 oz. portion) in the temperature normalizing process. Thus, the net calorie loss per ounce of beer is 1,020 calories. It doesn't take a rocket scientist to calculate that 12,240 calories (12 oz. x 1,020 cal./oz.) are extracted from the body in the process of drinking a can of beer. Frozen desserts, e.g., ice cream, are even more beneficial, since it takes 83 cal./gm to melt them (i.e. raise them to 0 deg. C) and an additional 37 cal./gm to further raise them to body temperature.

The results here are really remarkable, and it beats running hands down. Unfortunately, for those who eat pizza as an excuse to drink beer, pizza (loaded with latent calories and served above body temperature) induces an opposite effect. But, thankfully, as the astute reader should have already reasoned, the obvious solution is to drink a lot of beer with pizza and follow up immediately with large bowls of ice cream. We could all be thin if we were to adhere religiously to a pizza, beer and ice cream diet.

Protein

In 1838, Professor G. J. Mulder wrote, "There is present in plants and in animals a substance which is without doubt the most important of all the known substances in living matter, and, without it, life would be impossible on our planet. This material has been named Protein." Protein comes from the Greek word *proteios* for primary or "of the first rank." Professor Mulder's statement tells us why a word meaning primary was chosen.

Compared to proteins, carbohydrates and fats are nothing but logs (logs, after all, are just straight sticks of fuel). Proteins are long, curled, twisted and bent chains of small molecules called amino acids. Amino is the chemist's term for anything that has an atom of nitrogen in it. There are about two dozen amino acids and most have Greek or Latin names. For example, tyrosine is an amino acid found in cheese so you won't be surprised when I tell you tyrosine comes from a Greek word meaning cheese.

Most proteins are very large but there are some that have only a few amino acids. The small proteins are called peptides, probably because they are so small and full of pep.

The language of proteins is not nearly as confusing as the lipid language. Things whose names end with "ase" are enzymes. Except for base, case and erase. I've sometimes wondered if the 'ase' in enzymes didn't come from erase because once a substance is attacked by an enzyme, it's rubbed out. Enzymes are proteins that make things happen and happen very, very fast in our bodies. Enzymes either put things together or take them apart, like ministers in the chapel and judges in the divorce court.

There are thousands of enzymes but I'll discuss just a few so you get a good feel for the naming system. Sucrase breaks down sucrose (common table sugar) into glucose (blood sugar) and fructose (fruit sugar). Lactase is a fairly well known enzyme. It breaks down the carbohydrate in milk called lactose. People whose lactase enzyme is missing or malfunctioning get awfully gassy and spend a lot of time going to the loo after drinking milk. I've been told it's a crappy experience, a lot like eating food made with olestra.

Another enzyme is called tyrosinase. It breaks up the amino acid tyrosine and puts it into a substance called melanin. Melanin is the pigment that makes our skin darken and protects us from the ultraviolet rays of the sun. Humans and animals that don't make tyrosinase are albinos. Luckily, tyrosinase is not found in cheese, otherwise the cheese would turn black.

Lipase is an enzyme used to make lips. Birds don't have this enzyme; that's why they lack lips. Seriously, lipase breaks up long chains of lipids. There is no cellulitease or somebody would surely market it as the enzyme that "melts" the fat after you spend hundreds of dollars massaging those ugly lumps on your thighs.

Catalase is an enzyme used in butchering cattle. It's also an important antioxidant. There are two enzymes named for women, amylase and esterase. The former chews up starch in the stomach and the latter tacks a special chemical onto proteins that have overstayed their welcome in cells, marking them for destruction.

Not all proteins are enzymes. Proteins do just about everything. A story titled "The Perils of Proteus" best illustrates the variety of jobs performed by proteins.

A young man named Proteus Bold stopped at a shop to buy a cup of coffee and a danish on his way to work. A man named Elmer Coli who couldn't understand why business wasn't better at "E. Coli's Food Emporium" recently opened the shop. Proteus was standing at the counter of the nearly deserted shop when he noticed a woman, whose looks could start an avalanche, seated in a nearby booth. The keratins **(hair)** on her head were straggly and hadn't been washed for a week. Her **nail** keratins had been painted with polish obtained from a slashed artery. She was so skinny one would refer to her as collagen and collagen (**skin** and **bones**). Elastin (**blood vessels**) poked out from her arms.

"God," Proteus muttered, "that woman is ugly."

Seeing whom he was looking at, the equally ugly person standing beside Proteus said, "That's my girlfriend," as he raised a clenched fist. The man hadn't bathed or brushed his teeth for a while, which activated our hero's olfactory receptors (**smell**).

Proteus's rods and cones (**sight**) and organs of Corti (**hearing**) took this all in, sending distress messages to the brain, "Houston, we've got a problem." The brain sent a quick telegram to a couple of glands sitting on the kidneys wrapped in globs of fat. The glands immediately dumped a load of adrenalin **(hormone)** into the blood. The adrenalin rushed to actin and myosin (**muscles**) and liver to kick start the apparatus needed to defend Mr. Bold.

Having determined that the man threatening Proteus was endowed with growth hormone (**hormone)**, the brains cells **(memory)** decided the best course of action was to cut and run. Proteus grabbed his coffee and danish (mostly carbohydrate and fat) and threw a bill on the counter. His actin and myosin (**muscles**), fueled by stored carbohydrates and spurred into action by adrenalin (**hormone**) carried him quickly across the store and out the door.

Outside and safe from his avenger, Proteus gulped down the danish and swigged some coffee. His gustatory receptors (**taste**) sent a contented message to his brain while some enzymes (**digestion**) shared the danish down in the intestines. Fats from the sweet roll were carried out of the intestine on lipoproteins (**transport**) as insulin (**hormone**) rushed out of the pancreas to combine with receptors (**internal cell communication**), which reminded the cells to provide escorts (**cell transport**) for the glucose when it arrived.

While Proteus was waiting for his bus, a mugger poked a knife into his ribs and demanded his wallet. The brain and adrenalin did their thing again, enabling our hero to wrench the knife away and send the robber fleeing. Proteus cut himself in the struggle but proteins (**blood clotting**) immediately went to his rescue and saved him from bleeding to death. The wound didn't hurt much because endorphins and enkephalins (**pain killers**) were rushed to the brain.

The bus was crowded when Proteus climbed aboard so he was forced to stand, along with several others. Several people beside him were sneezing or coughing, spewing rhinovirus into the atmosphere. Seeking another body in which to take up residence, a million viruses found their way through Proteus's nasal passage and began dispersing. A passing gammaglobulin (**immune response**) noted the influx of the foreigners and immediately alerted the immune system. His blood was soon packed with an immunoglobulin army (**immune response**), which attacked and destroyed the invading rhinos.

Upon arriving at work, Proteus had barely sat down at his desk when a coworker rushed up to tell him the owner of the company had died and the son would become CEO. No sooner had the coworker finished the story than the ugly couple from E. Coli's strolled into the building. "Who's that?" came the whispers.

"The son," somebody replied. "Our new boss."

The adrenalin (**hormone**) level of several women went up, increasing their heart (**muscle**) and respiration (**muscle** and **transport**) rates and they fainted.

Proteus resigned and is now working as a clerk for a law firm that specializes in suing companies that manufacture or sell food products that make people fat (a.k.a. lipid).

Before leaving the subject of proteins, a *caveat emptor* story. Several years ago, a lady called me at home and began a sales pitch for superoxide dismutase (**antioxidant**). SOD had been discovered a few years before and was shown to be one of the antioxidants made in the body so I listened with interest. The marketer told me she was selling a supplement that contained SOD. This supplement, she claimed, would help prevent aging and also prevent several diseases. What she said about antioxidants was true but her product was a fraud.

"Are you aware that SOD is a rather large protein?" I asked.

"Yes, but our manufacturing process has managed to get it into a capsule," she replied.

"Proteins are completely broken down into their constituent amino acids in the stomach and small intestine," I explained. "Your SOD would never reach the blood."

There was a long silence before she countered, "But the amino acids will go to wherever SOD is made and make a brand new one."

"The chances of that happening are as likely as you winning the lottery," I said.

Similar scenarios are taking place today with human growth hormone. Touted as a supplement that will stimulate muscle growth and restore your body to that of a teenager, HGH is a protein made up of 191 amino acids. It is not a small protein and will be denatured in the stomach and completely digested in the intestines. The amino acids from the oral growth hormone will not go to a specific synthesis site and be converted back into the original. If that could occur, diabetics could use oral insulin.

The Vitamins

The word vitamin was unheard of before 1911, but 1500 years before the birth of Christ people knew that simply feeding a sick person a particular food could cure certain diseases. Early scientists who searched for the mysterious substances in food would have found nothing funny about nutrition. These men and their writings were ridiculed and harassed by contemporary scientists for believing there were certain unknown elements that were sometimes absent in the best of diets. The worst was they were unable to determine the composition of those unknown ingredients. While foods contain large quantities of carbohydrates, fats and proteins, vitamins are present in minute amounts, making them difficult to isolate and identify. Despite the scorn heaped upon them, several pioneers persevered and eventually succeeded.

Near the beginning of the 20th Century, Frederick Hopkins stated that foods contain a small amount of "growth factors" needed to sustain growth and life itself. The growth factors were defined as (1) substances found to be absolutely necessary for life (vital) and which (2) the body cannot synthesize on its own.

Several years after Hopkins published his beliefs about the unidentified growth factors, a Polish-born chemist named Casimir Funk successfully isolated a growth factor from rice husks. Funk said that the growth factors should be called "vitamines" because they were required for life (vita) and because he found that the substance he'd isolated contained nitrogen (amine).

Following Funk's success, there was a flurry of activity with vitamin research and some confusing Greek names started cropping up. Scientists interested in vitamines decided to have a meeting so the name game wouldn't get out of hand.

At the meeting, one of the scientists stood up and said, "carbohydrate, fat and protein nomenclature is laborious and confusing. I suggest we give the vitamines simple names that students and professors can remember and pronounce." The idea was accepted amid thunderous applause.

After some discussion and voting, the scientists decided to name the vitamines with letters of the alphabet in order of discovery. They named a substance not made in the body and needed to prevent blindness and keep their wives' skin soft vitamine A but then somebody reminded them Dr. Funk's vitamine had been discovered earlier. Following some deliberation, the scientists decided Casimir wouldn't mind so they stayed with their first decision. Retinol became vitamine A, and Funk's vitamine was named B.

The scientists were happily smoking their pipes and tacking on alphabetical names when somebody yelled, "Whoa! Back up here. There are only twenty-six letters in the alphabet. How do we know there aren't more than twenty six vitamines?" This was met with much consternation and deliberation until a decision was made to use subscripts with each of the letters beginning with B. Dr. Funk's vitamine was renamed vitamine B_1 and the meeting went on. A few years later at another meeting, the scientists dropped the subscript system when they figured there would be enough letters in the alphabet. By the time of that meeting, vitamines B_1, B_2, B_3, B_5, B_6 and B_{12} were the only B vitamines to pass muster. B vitamines four, seven, eight, nine, ten and eleven were discarded as not meeting the criteria. And so it was in 1935 the antiscurvy vitamine was called simply vitamine C.

After scientists identified, purified, and synthesized all of the vitamins, there was another big meeting where the attendees learned many of the vitamines do not contain nitrogen. The scientists decided to change Funk's original term "vitamine" to vitamin. Also, it was announced that a couple of the vitamins, vitamin D and B_5, can actually be made in the body but not in the amounts necessary to maintain health. They also decided to classify the vitamins as either water-soluble, if they floated around in the blood all day, or fat-soluble if they ended up in gobs of lipid (the correct term for fat) in and around body organs.

Funk might have screwed up with his name proposal but we have to admire Casimir for what he didn't do. Back in the days when there was a frenzy to name newly discovered stuff, many scientists attached their own names to their discoveries. Dr. Corti named a glob in the ear that makes hearing possible the organ of Corti. A scientist studying the pancreas found some unusual cells and named them after his family, thus we have the Islets of Langerhans (remember, these are in the pancreas not the Caribbean). Had ol' Cas decided to tack his name onto his discovery, we'd have water-soluble Funks and fat-soluble Funks. Because of his Polack humility we've been spared Funk A, Funk B_6. Funk C or Funk E. Another topic studied in nutrition along with vitamins is minerals. If the namer of vitamins had used his name and the namer of minerals was Wagnal, nutrition students would study Funks and Wagnals.

Fickle individualists they are, scientists nowadays use a combination of the alphabet system and Greek or Latin names, and for no apparent reason. Ask a nutritional scientist or biochemist to give you the name of vitamin B_1 and they'll look at you like you like you're drooling sewer foam. Thiamin is now the accepted name for B_1; B_2 is riboflavin and B_3 is niacin. Vitamin B_6 is, amazingly, vitamin B_6 and vitamin B_{12} is most often called vitamin B_{12}. The incongruity has nothing to do with complex names; B_6 is pyridoxine and B_{12} is cobalamin. A name couldn't be much simpler than retinol but it's most often called vitamin A. Admittedly, cholecalciferol (vitamin D) and alpha-tocopherol (vitamin E) are a little long winded but are they really that bad? Phylloquinone is a bit much so vitamin K definitely works better here. Ascorbic acid (vitamin C) is on the fence. Professionals trying to sound scholarly and sophisticated tend to use ascorbic acid while most lay folks refer to it as vitamin C.

Fat-soluble Vitamins

When all was said and done, the fat-soluble vitamins (A,D,E,K) turned out to be a big surprise. Unlike the water-soluble vitamins that most often work with enzymes—themselves water soluble—fat-soluble vitamins had nothing to do with enzymes. Two of the fat-solubles turned out to be antioxidants (A and E), vitamin D is actually a hormone and vitamins A and K act like they are. Hormone is derived from the Greek (are you surprised?) verb *hormao* meaning to excite or arouse. Hormones start metabolic events that would otherwise remain at rest.

If you're wondering what happened to vitamins F through J, wonder no more. They were never discovered and were never discarded. After vitamin E, the alphabet soup was ignored and vitamin K was named for the Danish word *koagulation,* meaning to clot.

Fish oils contain a lot of the fat-soluble vitamins. Many of those reading this book can probably remember when Mom poured a teaspoon full of cod-liver oil and made us gag it down. Thank God for food fortification and supplements.

Vitamin A

According to some nutrition texts, "Vitamin A was the first of the accessory food factors to be identified as a component of specific foods." (Oops!) It was a couple years after Dr. Funk identified a vitamine in rice hulls that two scientists fed rats a yummy diet consisting of carbohydrate, protein, lard and salts (for taste, no doubt). The rats didn't grow (go figure) so the scientists threw some eggs and butter into ether, stirred the mess, threw away what was left of the eggs and butter and let the ether evaporate. The stuff that was left after the ether evaporated (it's called an ether extract) was added to the carbohydrate, protein, lard and salt meal and fed to rats (I hope I wasn't a white rat in my former life). The rats grew which proved that the substance extracted from the eggs and butter was fat-soluble. Before the big naming meeting, it was called the fat-soluble growth factor. Also, some scientists discovered that rats forced to eat diets lacking the butter and eggs extract became blind (this was long before animal rights activists).

George Wald, a biochemist at Harvard, discovered how vitamin A works in the eye. His efforts were rewarded with the Nobel Prize in physiology or medicine in 1967. Shortly after receiving the award, Wald was invited to dinner by representatives of the U.S. Department of Defense. Over cigars and cognac, the government representatives asked their guest to help develop chemicals that could be used as blinding agents in chemical warfare. Furious, Wald poured cognac into their laps, picked up another cigar and left in a huff.

The primary job of vitamin A is in the visual process (you can see why it's such an important vitamin). However, vitamin A is also an antioxidant, it promotes growth and it keeps the skin and linings of blood and intestinal vessels from getting too rough and scaly. The last two are the hormone actions of the vitamin.

Elephant, rhino and elk horns grew because vitamin A is forbidden from entering horny cells. Automobile and truck horns are made from metals that don't contain vitamin A. In my opinion, one of the mysteries of science will always be the carrot. Carrots are a rich source of vitamin A but "smooth as a baby's behind" doesn't describe the skin of a carrot.

Vitamin D

Vitamin D is a vitamin only because of some clever persuasion. Before deciding on the absurdity of that statement, hear me out. Back in the 17th century, two different scientists described a medical problem that came to be known as rickets. People with rickets have soft, very weak bones—the legs are usually bowed because the bone isn't strong enough to support the weight of the body. In the early 1920s an English scientist was working with dogs that developed the bone disease described hundreds of years earlier. Influenced by the burgeoning interest in nutritional science, the scientist tested some different diets and discovered that cod liver oil was an excellent food additive for preventing rickets (Moms have known that since antiquity). The English scientist suggested that the substance in the cod liver oil was similar to vitamin A.

Either the lure of discovering a vitamin obstructed the Englishman's reasoning processes or he wasn't very observant because he apparently never considered the environment in which his experimental animals had been reared. The dogs were raised exclusively indoors (no sunlight and no ultraviolet light)!

Scientists on this side of the Atlantic finally solved the puzzle of the enigmatic "vitamin." First, a team of researchers at the University of Wisconsin showed that vitamin A was not the substance responsible for preventing rickets. Then another team, more observant than our English friend, irradiated skin with sunlight or ultraviolet light and showed that a substance that could prevent rickets was produced. Finally, two researchers raised some rats in the dark, causing them to develop rickets. They then irradiated some skin and fed it to the rats with rickets (you read right, they fed them skin). The skin supplement cured the rickets. It's fortunate we were able to identify vitamin D and mass produce it. Skin supplements would have never caught on.

When the time came to tack a name onto "the stuff that prevents rickets," a great debate ensued. On one side of the aisle scientists argued, "there's a great deal of interest in vitamin research these days and Congress is allocating money for vitamin research so let's call the substance a vitamin." From the other side of the aisle came the argument, "the substance is made in the body and has all the properties of a hormone, therefore it is a hormone."

"Sunshine hormone doesn't have the same marketing appeal as sunshine vitamin."

"But it's a hormone, in fact, it's a steroid hormone!"

"I love it when you talk dirty."

"Hormones don't come from the diet."

"What about passion fruit?

"How about we make a trade?"

"Do you think consumers are going to want to hear their milk is fortified with hormones?"

"You give us the rickets thing and we'll give you growth hormone. That should be an easy sell."

"Go fish."

The debate went on into the wee hours of the morning but in the end when the final vote was taken (it's amazing how many scientific discoveries have been put to a vote) a steroid hormone was classified as a vitamin and named vitamin D.

For your edification:

The nutritional scientists really deprived the endocrinologists (Ists who study hormones) of a complex, nomadic hormone. When you take a stroll through the park (but not down a lane where it's dark) or frolic on the beach, that horrific killer substance called cholesterol gets a sun tan. From the skin our substance goes first to the liver and then to the kidneys for a makeover before heading off to work in the intestines where it directs the construction of calcium transport proteins. These are called simply calcium binding proteins. They're needed to transport the calcium from your milk and cheese into the blood. Scientists considered naming them Cal Trans but the California Department of Transportation already had that one.

After punching the clock in the intestines, our peripatetic director of operations rushes off to its second job in the bones where it oversees the recruitment of calcium from the blood for bone building. The reason or need for the circuitous path taken by vitamin D to perform its role in the absorption and utilization of calcium remains a mystery but Mother Nature gets her jollies from mystifying scientists. She must have gotten a real belly laugh when the humans called her hormone a vitamin.

If our Mother Nature directs activities on planets in other galaxies, she probably has vitamin D in the creatures on the planet Hhemroyd going directly from the skin to the intestines and bones while insulin starts out from the stomach after a meal, travels to the lungs for a breath of fresh air and then goes to the pancreas before setting out on its mission to the muscles and fat cells.

There is some dissension among the professional ranks as to just how much U.V. light is needed to turn the "sunshine vitamin" into a working thing. Some claim a short walk from the main office building to the parking lot is enough as long as the sun is shining. Others think one needs to streak the entire length of the Las Vegas strip, buck naked in broad (no pun intended) daylight in order to convert the slovenly cholesterol into a sprightly hormone.

Vitamin E

Long before Viagra came on the scene, we had vitamin E. During some of the early experiments with vitamin E, scientists noted that rats fed diets deficient in this fat-soluble vitamin failed to develop sexually. Some unscrupulous marketers took advantage of this discovery and began touting vitamin E as a substance that would improve sexual virility. To this day, vitamin E is sometimes advertised as the sex vitamin but there appears to be no real evidence for any improved sexual vitality using vitamin E. That is why old fart celebrities endorse the V that ends in A rather than E.

Aside from turning male rats into stud muffins, the most important job of vitamin E is keeping the PUs in our PUFAs. If you recall, PUFAs are polyunsaturated fatty acids. They are some of the most important chemicals in our cells. They're unsaturated because some carbon atoms forgot to pick up their share of hydrogen ions so a neighbor had to share in order to keep the fat chain together. They're polyunsaturated because a female chemist said so. Also "poly" (from the Greek for "a whole bunch") means many. The bonding (isn't that sweet?) in the unsaturated fats is constantly being harassed by some left-wing chemicals that had formerly been incarcerated. They're called free radicals. They come from dysfunctional chemicals and constantly try to break up Poly and the Unsaturates. Vitamin E hangs out with the group and rousts the radical bullies whenever they threaten any of the unsaturated couples. Because a breakdown in the link between unsaturated carbons spells disaster for a cell, vitamin E is a very important antioxidant bodyguard.

Professionals who specialize in witty ditties have called vitamin E "the vitamin looking for a disease." One of the controversies in nutritional science is whether or not it has found that disease. Several years ago, the Shute brothers in Canada noted that vitamin E helped prevent heart disease. Their work was ignored and medical journals refused to publish their results so the two physicians published their own journal and wrote books about their amazing results with vitamin E. Their studies were scorned and criticized but few comments were made when a study involving 48 patients found no beneficial results with vitamin E and supposedly laid the subject to rest. The Shute brothers and many others have persisted and today vitamin E is recognized as an important nutrient necessary for the prevention of heart disease.

Vitamin K

Like vitamin D, vitamin K narrowly missed becoming a hormone. Following the discovery that a fat-soluble substance is responsible for blood clotting, a naming meeting was organized in the Halls of Science. The substance, many argued, is a hormone because it initiates the clotting process and it's made in the body. The majority was ready to rule in favor of hormonal status until somebody bothered to ask where in the body it was made. "The intestines," came the reply.

"What part of the intestine?"

Following some hemming and hawing and clearing of the throat: "The bacteria in the intestines."

Reluctant to classify the flora and fauna residing in our guts as a body organ, the majority voted in favor of vitaminhood for the new substance. When the Dane who discovered the clotting factor (he was truly a great Dane) stood up to speak nobody could understand him and assumed he wanted his name, Dam, attached. They wanted no part of a Dam vitamin. An interpreter finally convinced the shouting mob the Dane was suggesting the name "vitamin K" for the reason I already mentioned.

Water-soluble Vitamins

With the exception of vitamin C, the important water-soluble vitamins belong to the B complex (thiamin, riboflavin, niacin, B6, B12, folic acid, pantothenic acid, biotin, choline, inositol and PABA). The term "B complex" is a misnomer because each of the B vitamins does its own thing. The name came about because the B vitamins work together and they're often found in the same foods such as honey, which is nothing more than bee puke.

All of the B vitamins join with some kind of an enzyme to make things work quickly and efficiently, particularly in the nervous system which controls just about everything that goes on inside us. The Bs also help to repair the everyday wear and tear on our cells and they keep the immune system pumping out the tools of war needed to do battle with invading organisms. At the risk of having this book banned by the American Dietetic Association (ADA), the RDAs for the B vitamins are woefully inadequate.

Biotin, choline, inositol and PABA (para-amino benzoic acid is way more information than you need) are not essential because we make them in our bodies. Then why are they called vitamins? Probably part of the vitamin D deal. Choline and inositol help prevent fat accumulation in the liver. Now if we could just convince them to take up residence in our thighs, tummy and butt. Biotin helps prevent hair loss but (sorry, guys) doesn't help prevent baldness. PABA prevents graying of hair in rats but not humans (Mother Nature up to her old tricks again).

The F word

Several years ago Dr. Philip Handler, then President of the National Science Foundation (NSF), was called before a U.S. Senate Committee to discuss the Foundation's proposed budget. During the course of the hearings, one of the Senators remarked, "I hear you biochemists want to adulterate bread by adding vitamin B to it. If the good Lord had wanted vitamin B in bread He would have put it there."

Dr. Handler replied, "The good Lord did put vitamin B in bread. It was man who took it out in order to make white bread. The scientists who want to put it back are doing God's work."

A conservative, southern Senator had heard about the proposed fortification of bread and milk from an aide. "I don't care what those perverts do with bread and milk in their laboratories," he snarled at the aide, "I won't have any of that going on in public while I'm a Senator."

Thiamin and Brimstone

Back in the mid-1800s, eating polished white rice became all the rage in Far East. Soon after the inhabitants of those countries eliminated the brown-hulled grains from their diets, a frightening disease spread through the land. Medical experts and other sages of that era were sure an infectious plague was threatening the populace. Although the new disease—called beriberi—appeared along with the trendy practice of excluding brown rice, very few recognized the connection and white rice remained the socially acceptable thing to serve.

First sister to second sister (in Japanese, of course), "Oh gross! You're still eating that brown rice!"

Second sister to first sister (also in Japanese), "Is there something wrong with brown rice?"

First sister to second sister (in Japanese), "It's, like, totally unacceptable. Nobody, like, eats brown rice anymore."

Second sister to first sister (more Japanese), "I do."

In the midst of the polished rice craze, a young Japanese medical officer (the husband of the first sister who had recently been hospitalized because of swollen limbs and weak muscles) was sitting in his study when a servant brought him a bowl of polished rice. After studying the bowl a moment, the medical officer had a brilliant idea. He had a swig of Sake, left the uneaten rice and rickshawed to his headquarters where he asked for permission to conduct an experiment.

A few weeks later, two ships headed for the high seas. The galley of one ship was filled with the usual seafood: rice (polished, of course, since seamen were trendy), some vegetables and fish. The second vessel's larders contained wheat, milk, meat and unpolished rice.

When the two ships returned to port, the young medical officer was given immediate genius status. The experiment was a resounding success. The crew of the first ship was ravaged by beriberi; twenty-five seamen died. The survivors' reaction was, "#$@*&%&#!"

There were no symptoms of beriberi and no deaths on the second ship. The Japanese Admiralty quickly adopted a new diet for the entire navy. The medical officer published his findings, which were quickly scorned, criticized and disregarded.

Working on the island of Java—where beriberi was rampant—a young Dutchman had been watching some odd acting chickens. The birds scurried around holding their heads as if they were listening for worms. The Dutchman was smart enough to know chickens don't eat worms, which made him suspect the poor creatures were infected with beriberi like most of the human population. Miraculously though, those same chickens didn't die and even stopped listening for worms. The Dutchman pondered and probed, wandered and wondered, studied and scanned until he finally realized the chickens listening for worms had been eating polished rice but stopped their silly behavior when given brown rice.

The Dutchman made a trip around the island talking to the natives and making notes. He soon discovered that the islanders who remained healthy ate only brown rice while those who collapsed from muscle weakness and swelling ate the more chic polished rice. He conducted experiments to show that eating unpolished rice could cure people suffering from the dreaded disease. His observations were dismissed as "too simple to believe" but the Dutchman persisted and eventually our good friend Casimir Funk found "an amine vital for life" in the hulls of rice. I'm at a complete loss as to why the vitamin was named thiamin, originally thiaxnine. *Thi* is from a Greek word meaning brimstone but I fail to see the connection.

Poor People's Disease

The second infectious disease to be laid to rest by a vitamin was pellagra. In Italian (that's a switch) *pellagra* means "rough skin." That explains a person's appearance, but the disease is far more disastrous, eventually resulting in insanity and death. The disease most often occurred in poor rural families who lived primarily on corn and was referred to as corn poison or corn infection.

In the early 1900s, thousands of people died of pellagra in the United States alone. Because of its rapid spread, the United States Health Department sent Dr. Joseph Goldberger to the deep South, where the corn plague had reached epidemic proportions. The conditions Goldberger found were appalling. Victims of the disease were listless, slumped over and covered with blotches. Considering the poor hygiene—flies crawling everywhere—he easily could have been misled into believing the "infection" theory.

Goldberger, however, suspected that the cause of the disease could be traced to poor diets. He had visited state asylums where he noted that the patients developed pellagra but the staff did not. This was puzzling since there was frequent contact between staff and patients. In the dining rooms Goldberger saw the staff eating milk, meat, and eggs, while the patients lived mostly on cereals. Goldberger told the nation pellagra could be cured and prevented with adequate diets. Newspapers printed the results of his studies showing protein could eradicate pellagra.

Ignoring Goldberger's observations and pronouncements, a "specially appointed commission" published the view that pellagra was an infectious disease caused by the sting of the stable fly! Goldberger was horrified. He firmly believed that until nutrition was recognized as the cause of pellagra, people would continue to die by the thousands.

Goldberger came up with a plan that would convince the naysayers pellagra resulted from poor diet. After consulting with colleagues, he told the nation he and fifteen other volunteers, under medical supervision, would "infect" themselves by taking mucus from pellagra victims into their bodies. Skeptics thought Goldberger and his volunteers were fools but, to the astonishment of many, none of the volunteers developed pellagra. Goldberger's conclusions were accepted, and with dietary education the "infectious disease" known as pellagra was eradicated.

In the laboratory, Goldberger tried unsuccessfully to isolate and identify the substance that prevented the sickness he had successfully eliminated. He knew it was a substance in food but was unable to separate it from the other food components. In 1937, a scientist working with liver finally isolated the antipellagra factor.

Been there, done that

The antipellagra factor turned out to be a substance that chemists had known about for many years. It was a chemical called nicotinic acid. Imagine Dr. Goldberger's chagrin when he learned the substance he was unable to identify had been in a bottle on the shelf of every college chemistry lab in the United States. Also, when scientists discovered that nicotinic acid is made in the liver and kidneys, it nearly lost its vitamin status until it was determined most folks can't make quite enough to keep them completely healthy.

Since the antipellegra vitamin was nicotinic acid, nicotinic acid was destined to become a vitamin but that was not to be. The same conservative southern Senator who tried to block food fortification but failed saw a way to gain some measure of respect when he was told nicotinic acid was going to be added to bread and milk. Even though many of his constituents raised tobacco, he was sure they wouldn't want some chemical made from nicotine added to their food. Another Senator argued folks might think they could get the vitamin from cigarettes or cigars. The scientists were told to forget adding nicotinic acid to food so they did the only thing they could, they changed the name. Thus, nicotinic acid in the chemistry lab is nicotinic acid and when the liver produces the chemical it's nicotinic acid but when it behaves like a vitamin or gets added to bread and milk it's niacin. The name (I'm almost positive) was derived as follows: **Ni**cotinic acid **ac**ting as a vitam**in.**

Could somebody have been wrong?

The saga of niacin doesn't end with the naming scam. There is a strong possibility Dr. Goldberger was right for all the wrong reasons or scientists misinterpreted his ideas. After visiting the "poor folks" in the South, Dr. Goldberger recommended that they eat a variety of foods containing protein. He either suspected their corn-rich diets lacked some of the amino acids needed to stay healthy or he thought a vitamin was missing from the diets or perhaps both. As stated above, nicotinic acid is made in the liver and kidneys. This occurs along a biochemical disassembly line (the antithesis of Mr. Ford's idea) that tears the limbs off an amino acid called tryptophan. The fragmentation of tryptophan has a fork where one path leads to nicotinic acid and the other leads to a substance called picolinic acid.

This author and several others have shown that picolinic acid is a metal transporter. It goes into the intestine and swims around in the swill until it finds a metal ion. Zinc is its favorite. Picolinic acid joins with a metal and transports it into the blood where it's picked up and used in biochemical machines.

In the late 1970s and early 1980s, Dr. Ingeborg Krieger was treating children who developed a disease characterized by a terrible skin rash, among other things. I won't make you read the long name of the disease or try to pronounce it. Suffice it to say, the disease resembles pellagra in many ways and Dr. Krieger noted this in her studies. This disease also shows all the characteristics of young children who don't get enough zinc in their diet. Zinc is needed for many biochemical operations and the children she was working with were definitely deficient in zinc even though their diets contained enough to keep other children healthy.

Dr. Krieger deduced that the children could not absorb zinc from their intestines after eating a meal. Hearing about picolinic acid, she contacted this author and together we discovered that the children under her care could not make picolinic acid. When we chemically combined zinc and picolinic acid and put it in the children's food they quickly recovered.

Because pellagra and zinc deficiency cause very similar problems,

Dr. Krieger has suggested that the antipellegra factor may be picolinic acid rather than niacin. Her reasoning goes back to Goldberger when he showed that adding a variety of proteins to an otherwise corn-rich diet prevented pellagra. Corn contains very little tryptophan so folks eating mostly corn make very little picolinic acid and absorb very little zinc. The fact that niacin supplements cure pellagra supports Dr. Krieger's theory: niacin supplements would allow all the tryptophan coming from the diet to be directed down the picolinic acid path because the liver and kidneys wouldn't have to make any niacin. Because pellagra is a forgotten malady, this debate may never be resolved but one has to wonder if niacin hasn't been highly overrated.

Vitamin C

The search for the cause of scurvy infection

Before 1970, vitamin C was known primarily as the vitamin that prevents the disease known as scurvy. Linus Pauling changed that with the publication of *Vitamin C and the Common Cold.* (Contrary to what many people think, Pauling did not discover vitamin C; he simply made it the most widely researched vitamin in history.) After the publication of Pauling's theories, researchers began actively investigating the vitamin. Today vitamin C is recognized—due to its action in the body as an antioxidant—as a very important substance for the prevention of several diverse diseases. While most people recognize vitamin C as a "superstar" among vitamins, few are aware that this important chemical was discovered as a result of a search for the cause of what was thought to be an <u>infectious disease</u>.

Put ashore to die

Sometime in the early 1700s, a ship set sail from England on a trading voyage across the Atlantic Ocean. As so often happened on sea voyages, one of the sailors became very ill. His gums were bleeding, his teeth were falling out, his skin was rough, brown, scaly and dry and his legs became so swollen the poor wretch could not stand or walk. The captain of the ship immediately recognized the symptoms as those of the ominous "scurvy infection." Realizing the ill-fated sailor was near death, the captain decided to put the man ashore on a deserted island in order to prevent spread of the "infection" to the remainder of the crew.

Crawling laboriously along the shoreline in search of some kind of nourishment, the marooned sailor began eating fresh grass from tufts sprouting up at the edge of the beach. Within a few days, the abandoned sailor was not only alive, he was able to stand and walk, albeit with some difficulty. Soon however, his strength and stamina returned and he was able to locate other sources of food.

The sailor survived on the desolate island until he finally managed to signal a passing ship. He probably would have been rescued earlier but with his long hair and beard and his crawling, he looked from a distance like a goat grazing along the beach. The captain sent a crew to the island to rescue the abandoned sailor. Imagine the disbelief among the rescuing crew when the obviously healthy sailor explained the circumstance of his marooning.

"Hey, mates," one exclaimed, "this bloke claims 'e's 'ad the scurvy infection and didn't die!" Loud roars of laughter followed.

Any doubts about the validity of the sailor's story were removed when the man was returned to his native England where he met and greeted former shipmates. The men who had been with the sailor when he was put ashore regarded the sailor with awe and the story of his resurrection soon spread throughout the docks of London.

One of those who heard the story and became intensely intrigued was the Scottish surgeon, Dr. James Lind. Since he was serving with the British fleet, the Scotsman was acutely aware of the thousands of seamen who succumbed yearly to the ravages of scurvy. Hearing the story of the sailor who "ate grass like a beast and lived," Lind began to wonder about the man's diet while aboard ship and after being deserted. During the voyage, the sailor developed the symptoms of scurvy, which disappeared after eating grass. Did the grass contain something not available from the galleys on board ship? Dr. Lind decided to conduct an experiment, which may have been the first clinical study in the history of nutrition.

Discovery and scorn

Dr. Lind first experimented in 1747 with patients who showed the symptoms of scurvy. To these diseased individuals he fed oranges and lemons. With a great feeling of discovery and accomplishment, the surgeon observed that the symptoms of scurvy disappeared within a few days after the affected men began eating the citrus fruits. In Dr. Lind's words, "the most sudden, and visible good effects were perceived from the use of the oranges and lemons; of those who had taken them being at the end of the six days fit for duty."

Rather than proclaiming the end of the scourge of scurvy, medical "experts" scorned and repudiated the idea that diet caused the disease. After all, the doubters decreed, the crews of some ships drank lemon juice and still succumbed to the dreaded disease. The skeptics failed to recognize the fact that lemon juice put aboard ships was boiled to preserve it—a preventive measure that turned out to be detrimental since boiling destroys vitamin C. Dr. Lind's monumental discovery was ignored for nearly fifty years while scurvy continued to be considered an infectious disease spread by some undiscovered contagion.

Convinced his preliminary observations were accurate and reliable, Dr. Lind continually cajoled the British Admiralty until they finally relented and allowed him to repeat his experiments. "Let the damn Scotsman do his experiments if it'll keep him from pestering me!" the head of the Admiralty shouted.

A fleet of ships set sail from England supplied with enough raw lemon juice to sustain the crews for a twenty-three-week voyage. Ordinarily a journey of this duration would have resulted in several cases of scurvy but no symptoms of the disease appeared. The fleet returned to port with healthy and jubilant seaman manning the ships.

The voyage planned by Dr. Lind differed from previous voyages only in that daily rations of raw lemon juice were given the men.

Otherwise, the crews were exposed to the same harsh shipboard conditions. The results of the experimental voyage were so spectacular lemon juice was made a primary ingredient of the regulation diet supplied to British seamen. Later, lemon juice was replaced with lime juice, which gave rise to the nickname "limeys" for British sailors and often British citizens in general.

Vitamin C is identified

Although James Lind's experiments with citrus fruits put an end to scurvy's mastery of the waves, one-hundred-forty-years elapsed before somebody discovered exactly what substance in selected foods prevents scurvy. By 1930 scientists had come to the realization that many foods contain substances other than protein, carbohydrate and fats that are necessary to sustain health. When attention was turned to the substance in fruits and vegetables that prevents scurvy, a Hungarian born chemist, Dr. Albert I. Szent-Gyorgyi, discovered vitamin C.

The man who isolated and identified vitamin C was both brilliant and colorful. Born in Budapest, young Szent-Gyorgyi entered the University of Budapest in 1911 as a medical student. He soon became bored with his studies and withdrew to join the Austro-Hungarian army in World War I. After being wounded while fighting on the Russian and Italian fronts, he resumed his studies and received his medical degree in 1917.

When the communists took over the Hungarian government after the war, Dr. Szent-Gyorgyi left Hungary to tour the world for 12 years, teaching in Germany, Holland, England (where he received a Ph.D. from Cambridge University) and the United States. In 1932 the government that overthrew the communists invited Dr. Szent-Gyorgyi to return to Hungary to work as a professor of medical chemistry and later a professor of organic chemistry at the university in Szeged. Following the Nazis' occupation of Hungary, Dr. Szent-Gyorgyi joined the resistance movement. Adolph Hitler ordered him captured and killed when he became aware Dr. Szent-Gyorgyi was delivering important scientific and political papers to the British.

While conducting experiments on cell respiration Dr. Szent-Gyorgyi succeeded in isolating a substance from plants that was effective in eliminating scurvy. While he was trying to unravel the exact structure of the substance Dr. Szent-Gyorgyi submitted a preliminary manuscript to a scientific journal in which he expressed his ignorance of the structure. He thought it was some kind of carbohydrate and, since the names of those compounds end in 'ose,' suggested naming it "ignose." Angered by the author's condescension, the editor of the journal rejected the paper. Dr. Szent-Gyorgyi quickly resubmitted the manuscript with a new proposed name, "godnose." Eventually the vitamin was appropriately named ascorbic acid because of its antiscorbitic action—scorbitic referring to diets resulting in the development of scurvy. In 1937, he received the Nobel Prize for physiology or medicine.

Dr. Szent-Gyorgyi's research was by no means limited to vitamin C. He also worked on cancer, muscle chemistry, problems relating to how the body produces and utilizes energy and the chemistry of the thymus gland. The American Heart Association honored him with the Lasker Award for his work studying the heart.

His research on the human body inspired his beliefs about mankind and the future of the human race. Angered by the U.S. presence in southeast Asia in 1966, Dr. Szent-Gyorgyi joined with other prominent persons in refusing to pay his income taxes to protest U.S. military forces in Vietnam and the Dominican Republic. The intriguing Hungarian often brought attention to serious problems by making unusual statements about them. In 1966, Dr. Szent-Gyorgyi warned of impending cannibalism unless the world population was controlled. His solution was for the U.S. government to disseminate birth control information to the world. In 1970, Dr. Szent-Gyorgyi complained, "We find out how nerves work and they make nerve gas; we find out how things grow and they make herbicides."

During the 1970s, his work concentrated on a theory that free electrons are a key in both the normal and abnormal behavior of human body cells. Such ideas, considered radical (those free electrons were later to become known as free radicals), often got his private and federal research funds cut off because he could not predict where his work would lead him. Today the free radicals Dr. Szent-Gyorgyi spoke of are considered one of the most prominent causes of disease in living systems.

"Discovery consists of seeing what everybody has seen and thinking what nobody has thought," is the quote most often attributed to Dr. Szent-Gyorgyi. My favorite however will always be, "When everyone begins to laugh at you, then you know you are two steps ahead."

Linus Pauling

No chronicle intended to annoy nutrition scientists would be complete without mentioning Dr. Linus Pauling, who to many in that field is a pariah or the "antichrist." Despite being the most celebrated and decorated chemist in history and the only person to ever win two unshared Nobel Prizes, the career of Linus Pauling was steeped in controversy. Pauling was an exceptional individual and some writers claim his gift of intelligence was responsible for the controversy that seemed to surround everything he did and everything he wrote. He was frequently criticized for the conclusions he drew from what some felt was too little experimentation, often outside of Pauling's area of expertise.

Although Linus Pauling eventually received a Ph.D. in Chemistry and 58 honorary doctorates, he never graduated from high school. The high school he attended in Portland, Oregon required their students to take a class in civics. Pauling saw no reason why he should attend the class. He figured he could learn the material on the streets and from his own reading. Later, after his Nobel Prize for Peace in 1962, the administration agreed that he had learned civics on his own so they granted him his high school diploma. Dr. Pauling assured the administrators the diploma would be helpful should he decide to seek employment in the future.

In the first of his important contributions to science, Pauling brought a specialized branch of physics (quantum physics) along with his powerful visual imagination into chemistry. Prior to his writings, chemical formulas had been presented as simple two-dimensional symbols in the pages of textbooks. Using the lengths and angles of the chemical bonds that hold atoms together, Pauling showed how to construct accurate three-dimensional configurations depicting the exact arrangement of atoms in a compound. Ordinary chemists, content with their science in its pre-Pauling cookbook stage, attempted to repel the intrusion of physics into their field. They not only resisted his conceptual argument and challenged his data, they called his integrity into question (the dissidents really wondered how a guy with no high school diploma could be so perceptive). Modern chemists, educated with textbooks that incorporate the revolution Pauling brought to the field of chemistry, would have difficulty understanding the rationale for that forgotten controversy. Pauling's early studies led to the eventual publication of "The Nature of the Chemical Bond," a landmark in the history of science.

In 1931, Pauling was awarded the Langmuir Prize of the American Chemical Society for "the most noteworthy work in pure science done by a man under 30 years of age." In the same year he was offered a joint full professorship in both chemistry and physics at the Massachusetts Institute of Technology (he only stayed a year because he didn't care for the winters in Massachusetts). Two years later, at the age of 32, he was made a member of the National Academy of Sciences, the youngest appointment to this body ever made. Can't you hear the stodgy old scientists grumbling about this appointment?

In the mid-1930s, Pauling turned his attention to working with biological molecules. For the next two decades he experimented with proteins to determine how they were arranged and how they functioned. While studying hemoglobin, Pauling discovered that sickle cell anemia is caused by a genetic defect leading to an abnormal structure. His studies with proteins led to the Nobel Prize for Chemistry in 1954.

During World War II Pauling, like everyone at Cal. Tech., worked on various "war" projects but he chose not to work on the development of the atomic bomb. I think he helped develop a great cannon for tanks, which is a little out of the realm of chemical bonds and proteins. Concerned about the radiation produced by the "bomb," Pauling became involved with a group of scientists working for safe control of nuclear power and was an outspoken opponent of nuclear testing and warfare. In 1947, President Truman awarded him the presidential Medal of Merit for his work on crystal structure, the nature of the chemical bond, and his efforts to bring about world peace.

In November of 1950, he was subpoenaed to appear before the Senate Investigating Committee on Education of the State of California. This was during the early days of the McCarthy "witch hunts" when you were accused of being a communist if you had a drink of vodka or stood beside somebody who did. Pauling was not nor had he ever been a communist or involved with the Communist Party. He did, however, fervently believe that no governmental body had the right to ask him to answer those questions under oath. His position upset some of the trustees and some professors at Cal. Tech., who tried to oust him.

In 1952, Pauling requested a passport to attend a meeting in England, to defend his theories about protein structures. The passport was denied. He applied again and wrote President Eisenhower, asking him to arrange the issuance of the passport since, "I am a loyal citizen of the United States. I have never been guilty of any unpatriotic or criminal act." After prolonged correspondence with the State Department, the passport was denied on the very day he was supposed to leave for the conference. Two years elapsed before Linus Pauling was allowed to travel abroad carrying a U.S. passport.

In 1954, Pauling was lecturing at Cornell University when he was called to the telephone to learn that he had just been awarded the Nobel Prize in Chemistry. He immediately applied for a passport to travel to Stockholm but heard nothing for several weeks. In Washington there was strong opposition to his application. The beleaguered passport was finally granted and arrived at his home barely two weeks before the ceremony in Sweden.

Another Nobel was in his grasp

The years of being unable to obtain a passport became far more than an inconvenience to Pauling. In 1948, he was already working toward a description of the structure of DNA. By the early 1950s, Rosalind Franklin and others working at Kings College in London possessed sharp, detailed photographs of the DNA molecule. James Watson and Francis Crick used these images in their successful discovery of the DNA double helix. Had Pauling been able to attend the spring 1952 conference he would likely have been shown the invaluable photographs and might have come to the same conclusion, before Watson and Crick. Not seeing the photographs contributed to his proposed structure which had the phosphate groups closely packed inside a single helix with the bases sticking out around the outside. Had it not been for his outspoken criticism of government policies, Linus Pauling, rather than Watson and Crick, likely would have been the author of "The Double Helix."

Pauling continued his political activism, particularly his protesting of atomic bomb testing. Public controversy, sustained by Pauling's forceful contributions, eventually induced the superpowers to suspend the testing of atomic bombs in the atmosphere. A treaty was signed and went into effect on the day of the bestowal of the Nobel Peace Prize for 1962 on Linus Pauling. This award was not universally popular. Many newspapers and magazines printed editorials denouncing him, his activism and his having been given the prize. He later received the Jehan Sadat Peace Award.

During the latter years of his career, Pauling focused on nutrition and the role of the micronutrients, especially vitamin C, in maintaining health. In 1970 he published a book for the lay reader, *Vitamin C and the Common Cold*, which received the Phi Beta Kappa Award as the best book on science of that year. Soon after, Pauling became interested in the use of vitamin C in the treatment of cancer, largely through his contact with the Scottish physician, Dr. Ewan Cameron. Their collaboration resulted in the 1979 book, *Cancer and Vitamin C*.

Until his death, Pauling continued to travel all over the world, lecturing on his classic work in chemistry, biology, medicine, and peace. Before his death, Pauling stated that he had come to believe the proper use of vitamin C and lysine can completely control, even cure, cardiovascular disease, heart attacks and stroke. Those who scorn Pauling revel in telling people he died of prostate cancer. They fail to mention he was 93.

Minerals

While the vitamins fostered countless heated debates as to their true origins, there never has been and never will be any doubt about the origin of minerals; they come from dirt. Unlike the vitamins with alphabet and ho hum Greek names, the minerals were named for gods and goddesses, important people and cities in New Jersey. Also, vitamins are mostly colorless but minerals have green, blue, red, violet, yellow, silver and gold hues. Some even ignite when scratched or explode when dropped into water.

Both vitamins and minerals are needed to keep the body going but there are some basic differences between the two. Vitamins are what chemists call organic. Organic is defined as anything that contains carbon. Coal and cyanide contain carbon but they're not considered organic so there are some exceptions.

Several years ago, J.I. Rodale, who was not a chemist, chose the term "organic" to describe foods fertilized with natural organic matter rather than chemical fertilizers, foods grown without application of pesticides and foods processed without use of food additives. Since organic applies to all things that contain carbon—except coal and cyanide—all foods are organic. Mr. Rodale was the publisher of *Prevention,* a magazine scorned and criticized by health professionals. Imagine the fun the "experts" had pointing out to Mr. Rodale that all foods are organic whether they've been fertilized with cow poop or some of Monsanto's potent poisons. Much ado about doo doo.

Another sidebar

During the past few years, pestaphobes (people who won't eat food grown with anything except dung) have been lobbying to have produce labeled as to just how much of the product is free of laboratory-synthesized fertilizers (as opposed to fertilizers produced in the large intestine of animals). The lobbyists want labels telling folks whether or not the food is "100% organic" or "95% organic." Unfortunately, there's a real problem here. As previously stated, all food is organic. That being a fact, an unscrupulous vendor could fill a bag with carrots or peas or collards—which are a kind of kale, which is like cabbage—that have been grown with all kinds of carcinogenic goodies and label the stuff as "100% organic." It would be, so an equally unscrupulous lawyer could defend the crooked vendor. I suggest they drop the term organic and use "pooduce." Thus, veggies grown exclusively with animal waste could be correctly and indisputably labeled "100% pooduce."

Just when the consumers of organically grown fruits and vegetables were feeling really smug about their healthy lifestyle, scientists discovered that these supposedly pesticide-free products in fact contain residues of long banned chemicals including DDT and chlordane. Although the food products were grown without the use of banned pesticides, plants can take up the chemicals because they remain in the soil for decades after being applied. Also, there are many special pesticides that have been approved for use on organically grown fruits and vegetables and recently some of them are now suspected of posing a cancer risk while others effect the brain. A food toxicologist from California recently stated, "Consumers need to recognize that organic production doesn't mean pesticide-free production." So, Mr. and Mrs. Smart Aleky, you're so pure, you're so pious, masticators of manure mulched multifolates you might be eating awful apples, cancerous carrots, contaminated cabbage, lethal leeks, poisonous peas, polluted pears, ravaged rutabagas, tainted turnips, toxic tomatoes, zapped zucchini or a whole bunch of other venomous vittles. Have a good day.

Back to Basics

Minerals contain no carbon. Minerals are "inorganic." Inorganic refers to anything that is not a plant or an animal. Inorganic can be confusing. When reading the sentence "minerals are inorganic," one might first think the sentence is incomplete. "In organic what?" you ask before realizing inorganic is one word. But why inorganic? Why not notorganic or nonorganic or ain'torganic?

The essentiality of minerals has been known since antiquity. Thousands of years ago the Chinese people would take a walk along the seashore and munch seaweed and sponge—good sources of iodine—if they felt an enlargement in their throat (goiter). Whenever the Greeks got that tired and run down feeling—anemia—they just dipped a heated sword into a mug of hot water and tossed back the concoction.

The minerals present a special set of problems. Minerals, after they're plucked from the earth, have a tendency to lose things, especially electrons. Despite their inability to keep track of their negative knick-knacks, they remain positive. It's that positive attitude that leads to problems.

Some foods contain chemicals that belong to the dastardly "ate" family—oxalate and phytate. Oxalate hangs out in spinach and other vegetables of that variety while phytate can usually be found in the whole grain saloon. Oxalate and phytate have a negative attitude. You've heard how opposites attract; oxalate and phytate manage to attract minerals that have lost some electrons with promises of ionic bonds.

Caly Cium to her father Cal Cium, "I'm like so attracted to Oxal Ate. I want to, like, go away with him."

"But Caly, he's so negative. Are you sure that's what you want?"

"I'm positive."

Once a mineral and an "ate" are joined together, they head off to the colon where their lives are wasted. The mineral never again sees its friends and relatives who are busy in the body working in important positions like bone builders, muscle contractors, supervisor of nerves, oxygen transporters and fat fighters.

A few of the essential minerals were unwittingly involved in one of the biggest scams in nutrition history—Popeye the Sailor cartoons, also known as the Spinach Spoof. In a typical episode, Bluto kidnaps Olive Oyl and carries her off on his boat. Popeye pursues but gets worn out in the process. When he confronts Bluto, the miscreant proceeds to beat Popeye senseless (there was a lot of violence and implied sex in that cartoon). In the course of the brawl, Olive Oyl manages to open a can of spinach and pour it down her hero's gut. Popeye suddenly jumps up, flexes his muscles and proceeds to pound Bluto into the ground. While Olive moons over her savior, Popeye sings his ditty about being strong to the finish because he eats his spinach.

The cartoon was obviously a scheme devised by frustrated parents who wanted their kids to eat their vegetables. The fact is, spinach contains a lot of oxalate and nobody, including Popeye, can squeeze the calcium out. If Olive's super stud had eaten spinach as regularly as he claimed, he would have become a wasted, brittle-boned village idiot. If the kids hadn't seen through the veiled attempt to make them healthy, nursing homes would be erected on every city block, packed with frail, anemic, broken-hipped wrinkled old geezers draining the Medicare and Medicaid coffers.

While most professionals agree spinach, and rhubarb pie for that matter, are poor sources of minerals there is some dissension about fiber and phytate. Whole grains and soy (more about this later) contain phytate but experiments don't seem to agree about whether or not the phytate causes a problem. To cover their fannies, professionals tell us to eat fiber but not too much. They, and therefore we, have no idea how much is too much. These same professionals also tell us to drink eight glasses of water a day; as we all know, water is made from two kinds of gin.

Some Mighty Minerals

Calcium

Make no bones about it (this phrase dates back to at least 1548 but God only knows its true origin), calcium is the most abundant mineral in the body. In addition to making strong teeth and bones, calcium is needed to make nerves work, it protects the heart and helps prevent some kinds of cancer. Because calcium is so important, we need a lot in the diet but the big debate is, where should we get it?

A reader asks, "What is the best source of calcium? I've read milk and other dairy products have a lot of calcium and it's easily absorbed, but milk and other dairy products have fat in them except for skim milk."

Expert's response: "Those milk-mustached hunks and hunkesses should all be taken down to the coulee and shot. Milk and other dairy products, including skim milk, which I call skam milk because they've taken out all the butt-bulging, thigh-thickening, gut-grossing fat—God, I miss it—is claimed to be healthy. But it's not. It's filled with hormones and pheromones and earphones and pesticides and fungicides and crimsontides and, in the winter, yuletides. In short, milk and other dairy products aren't good for you but I'm not sure why. More research is needed.

"Until then, eat lots, and I do mean lots, of vegetables. For example, although you can get the daily requirement, I can't remember if that's the RDA, U.S. RDA, RDI, DMV or DVM, for calcium from four glasses of milk, you only have to eat five cups of canned spinach; oops, forget that. You only have to eat four cups of collards, which are a kind of kale, which is like cabbage. If you're not into cabbage you'll have to eat about 30 cups of some kind of vegetable every day. Once in awhile you could substitute ten heads of lettuce in a day. That would give 50% of the daily requirement but that's close enough—you'll only break one hip if you fall—and you'll get a lot of that much needed dietary fiber to clean out the ol' colon. Roto Rooter in a leaf I call it.

"Keep those inquiries coming."

A caller asks, "Is it true calcium is absorbed best at night?"

Expert's response: "Not so fast. I've barely finished my cream-topped tofu pudding. Yes, I've read the studies suggesting calcium is absorbed best after dark. I haven't made up my mind as to their validly, more research is needed, but there may be some truth. The way I see it, after cholesterol gets sun burned and blinded by the UVs, the vitamin D goes to the liver until its eyes have gotten accustomed to the dark and then slips off to the kidneys to wait for sunset. When there's no more light shining on the kidneys, vitamin D schleps over to the intestines to start up the calcium transporter factory. The calcium transporters hang around in the intestines waiting for calcium. Some of the transporters will give up and go home if they aren't busy so it's best if there's calcium in the stomach in the wee small hours of the morning (sounds like a song doesn't it?). It certainly can't hurt to get your calcium before you go to bed so eat four cups of collards, which are a kind of kale, which is like cabbage or 30 cups of some other vegetable or ten heads of lettuce just before nodding off. Personally, I'd drink a glass of milk.

"Until next time, ta, ta."

While some experts are arguing for dairy products and others are pushing veggies as a source of calcium at least one expert claims the only form of calcium that is of any value comes from coral found in the East China Sea. According to a "world renowned bio-logical chemist" (I'd never heard of the man until I saw him on a late-night infomercial), coral calcium is where it's at. Back pain, fibromyalgia, diabetes and even cancer fade away when confronted by treatments of Sango Coral, which, according to the coral guru, contains an organic composition identical to that of the human skeleton. So, if you want to cure what ails you, book passage on a ship bound for Okinawa where you can lounge away the hours chomping coral. If you can't afford the trip, send $24.95 to some distributor who will be more than happy to ship you a supply of this clinically untested potion.

My book about chromium picolinate has been published in four languages. Does that mean I'm world renowned?

Sodium and Potassium

Sodium and potassium are known as electric lights. That's because when they're dissolved in water they can conduct an electric current. I mentioned earlier, minerals have a tendency to lose their electrons. When either sodium or potassium loses an electron it's attracted to chemicals that have too many electrons—opposites attract—and make salts. If you take a wire that has a current running through it, cut it and put the two ends into a glass of water with table salt dissolved in it, the water will continue to conduct the current and light the lights because the dissolved salt plays "hot potato" with the electrons coming out of one end of the wire, passing them back and forth until they arrive at the other end of the wire and go on their way (don't try this at home). On the other hand, if you took that same wire, cut it, put the ends in a glass of water and dropped in a pellet of pure sodium or potassium—no electrons lost—you'd blow the glass, the wire and yourself into the next county (definitely don't try this at home)!

Lucky for us sodium and potassium like to lose an electron. As I've illustrated, before they lose an electron these two are very explosive. Once they lose an electron they calm down. It's sort of like a frontal lobotomy. Consider the guy who profusely salts his eggs, hashbrowns, toast and ham before taking a bite. If the sodium in that table salt hadn't lost an electron so it could be salt, the guy's head would splatter brains or whatever for a city block as soon as the juices in his mouth touched the sodium.

Sodium and potassium along with calcium are the minerals that make our nerves work. Without them there would be no brain activity, no muscle activity, no organ function at all. I was once told by a female dietician that women are smarter than men simply because women retain salt.

Here's a little known fact, at least to the nonprofessional: the body needs about four times as much potassium as sodium. I won't go into the whys and wherefores; it has something to do with nerve function, elaborate mathematical formulas, the law of supply and demand and sine waves. Suffice it to say, nerves function optimally when there is four times as much potassium as sodium in the body. Having said that, I'll give you the bad news: it is difficult, not impossible, but difficult, to eat diets that have a four to one ratio of potassium to sodium. There is no good news unless you eat a lot of fruits and vegetables—good sources of potassium—and cut back drastically on your salt intake.

My wife makes an absolutely fantastic guacamole dip and guacamole is especially high in potassium. Now if we could just tolerate salt-free chips with her dip we could have a heart-healthy snack with our evening cocktails.

The atomic symbol for calcium is Ca, the atomic symbol for magnesium is Mg, the symbol for manganese is Mn (you're no longer wondering why magnesium isn't Ma), the symbol for hydrogen is H (Hy sounded too cheery), the symbol for oxygen is O (Oy sounded too Jewish) but the symbol for sodium (you were wondering where I was going with this) is Na and the symbol for potassium is K. While the symbol for most of the atomic elements is taken from the first, and many times a following letter in the name, the symbols for sodium and potassium were taken from their Latin derivatives, *natrium* and *kallium*. Take that with you to your next cocktail party.

Magnesium and Phosphorus

As with the other minerals, we're fortunate magnesium and phosphorus (P) lose some electrons before they enter our bodies. Pre-lostelectrons, these two are very combustible. One or both of these minerals are used in matches, fireworks, incendiary bombs and flares as well as various and sundry other products used to light up our lives.

After magnesium loses a couple of electrons so it won't burn or combust, it schleps into our bodies in food and supplements and begins performing a whole bunch of very important jobs. Biochemists have known for years that magnesium is essential and important but until recently didn't realize just how vital it is. Although scientists discovered early on that magnesium is used in the body to help many different enzymes and our cells wouldn't be able to produce enough energy without it, research during the last few years has shown that magnesium is necessary to prevent heart disease, stroke, diabetes, migraines and osteoporosis. But not bunions, boils and butt fungus. Those who do research with magnesium claim it is as important as calcium but those claims have to be taken with a grain of magnesium salt because these people depend upon grants to keep them in business. Nuts, wheat bran and wheat germ are good sources of magnesium but unless you eat about a quarter pound a day of these you need a supplement. Those studying to become Ists learn about the wheat and nuts but aren't told about the supplements.

For nutrition scientists, phosphorus is about as interesting as the chemical composition of pus. That's because phosphorus is found in every diet—high fat diets, low fat diets, medium fat diets, the Zone diet, Dr. McDougall's diet, the Mayo Clinic diet, the Grapefruit diet and even diets concocted by celebrities who don't know squat about nutrition. Phosphorus is everywhere so professionals don't worry and argue about it. There's phosphorus in the pages of this book, but please, don't eat them.

Phosphorus works with calcium to make strong teeth and bones. It's also used to make strong walls for cells. (Remember the phosphofats?) Without phosphorus, cells could not divide, the heart couldn't beat and the baby couldn't grow. Or cry for that matter.

I just realized I made an error. Sodium and potassium as well as calcium and magnesium are called electrolytes not electric lights. But I don't want to go all the way to the top of the chapter and change it.

More Minerals

Zinc

Zinc (Zn) was discovered to be essential in humans while Dr. Ananda Prasad was doing some research in Egypt. When young men in their early twenties visited his clinic, Dr. Prasad noticed that they were unusually small in stature for their age and one thing was particularly noticeable; they had tiny tally whackers. Dr. Prasad suspected iron deficiency so he gave the men iron supplements and sure enough, their ding-a-lings grew along with the rest of their bodies. Later, Dr. Prasad discovered that the iron supplements were contaminated with zinc so he tested some underdeveloped men with uncontaminated iron supplements and some with zinc. From these studies, scientists learned that zinc is needed for growth and development. I'll never forget attending a lecture at the University of North Dakota Medical School when a colleague of Dr. Prasad described the studies conducted in Egypt. Faces flushed throughout the auditorium as a vast array of before-and-after-zinc supplemented male genitalia appeared on the screen.

After scientists grew weary of observing wrinkled willies, they began looking at other parts of the body and learned that zinc is needed in every organ. Zinc is often referred to as the "intelligence mineral" because of the ion's crucial function in the implementation of the structural arrangement of protein catalysts located within the confines of the central and autonomic nervous system. Undoubtedly, if the person who coined the term "you are what you eat" had more zinc in the diet the phrase would be a much more recondite pleonasm: "The composition of the system of nerves, muscles and cells which undergo myriad multifarious metabolic reactions within the framework of said individual will without stipulation be a direct consequence of the composition of the animal, mineral and vegetable matter ingested by said individual."

Aristotle, Plato, Michelangelo and Einstein got a lot of zinc in their diets; most Congressmen, except those from North Dakota and Nevada, should use zinc supplements as should physicians who write advice columns for newspapers. People who talk on cell phones in restaurants or while driving also need a daily zinc supplement.

Zinc is needed for healthy skin, bones and hair. It is a part of enzymes used in digesting food and extracting oxygen from the air. Zinc is involved in removing carbon dioxide from blood, calcifying bone, manufacturing proteins and nucleic acids, development of the reproductive organs (do-dahs and such), healing wounds and tasting the food we eat. Zinc is needed in the immune system, in the prostate and in the eye. All this with a mineral that is used to galvanize nails and buckets before it loses a couple of electrons.

Health professionals tell us there is enough zinc in our food if we eat a balanced diet, but they're fibbing. Zinc is difficult to absorb from food because it needs a special transporter, picolinate, which is made from the amino acid tryptophan. Tryptophan is not a common amino acid in food so even if there is enough zinc in a food product, the body doesn't make enough picolinate to take all the zinc we need out of the food.

Selenium

Selenium is a mineral "rags to riches" story. It was discovered in 1817 but nobody paid it much attention. It didn't burn, glow, explode or galvanize nails but it did croak a lot of animals that were grazing on soils containing high amounts of the mineral. For years, selenium was considered a highly dangerous and toxic mineral until a scientist working at the National Institutes of Health discovered it would cure liver disease in rats. All over the world people were trying to exterminate rats when some goofy German scientist finds a way to keep them alive.

Following the report that selenium may be an essential mineral, the scientific literature was suddenly deluged with reports of sicknesses occurring in animals grazing on soils containing very little selenium. A paradox ensued; is selenium toxic to organisms or is it needed by organisms to sustain life? Yes to both. Scientists were reminded of the rule of Paracelsus, "the dose alone determines the poison," when they realized high doses of selenium stop the biochemical machines but low doses are needed to keep them operational.

One day, at a desk located in the Midwest, where the soil contains a lot of selenium, somebody discovered that the cancer rate was very low in that region although some horses, cattle and chickens got sick while grazing. More deskwork was carried out and many experiments were done after which scientists concluded that the low cancer rate was due to the high selenium content of the soil. Today selenium is recognized as one of the most important antioxidants in our diet.

Copper

Outside the body, copper (Cu) is used to make wire that carries current from giant complex electrical generators to our homes to power electric genital wart removers. Inside our bodies, sans a couple electrons, copper plays an important part in the production of the protein hemoglobin, which is vital for getting oxygen out of the air and into our cells.

It's trite but true, there's less copper in the human body than in a common penny. A little, however, goes a long way and copper is thought to help prevent heart disease and boost the immune system. Copper is part of an important antioxidant protein and it helps prevent arthritis (yes, copper bracelets can help).

Chromium

The same goofy German that kept the rats alive with selenium was working with another German scientist when they discovered they could make rats diabetic by feeding them a certain kind of yeast. Instead of buying stock in the company and announcing their discovery to the world so everybody could use the yeast to kill rats, they discovered another kind of yeast that would cure the diabetes. Being typical meticulous German scientists, the two assayed and analyzed until they realized the yeast that cured the diabetes contained chromium but the yeast that caused the diabetes didn't.

The only known job for chromium (Cr) in the body is to help the hormone insulin work effectively and efficiently. Chromium is difficult to absorb and it's nearly impossible to get enough from the diet. Beer and liver are good sources but you'd have to drink several gallons of beer a day to meet the demand. If you ate enough liver to get the chromium you need, you'd probably die from vitamin A toxicity. If you insist on getting your nutrients from grocery items, go to the health foods section of your local grocery store and purchase a supplement called chromium picolinate. Trust me.

FYI (these are shorter than sidebars): The chromium that made Erin Brockovitch rich and Julia Roberts even richer is completely different from the chromium that makes insulin work. The bad chromium has lost six electrons (no wonder it's so surly and contemptuous). It's called chromium 6. The good chromium has lost only three electrons—chromium 3—and is much more chivalrous.

Molybdenum

Molybdenum (pronounced moly-be-denum or if you want to get technical muh-lib-duh-num) is an essential part of tooth enamel. An American working with the U.S. Department of Agriculture showed that molybdenum decreased the incidence of dental caries in rats (the Germans saved them from liver disease and diabetes and the Americans worry about their dental health).

Molybdenum is a part of some important enzymes needed for metabolizing fat (there's an idea), carbohydrate and protein. According to Dr. K.V. Rajagopalan (not to be confused with Dr. V.K. Rajagopalan), molybdenum may help prevent birth defects.

Manganese

Manganese (Mn) was discovered by a woman, Dr. Carol Scheele, and a lot of the good research done with the mineral was performed by women. Here's a quote from a lady who has done a lot of work with manganese, "Biochemical reasons for the dermatitis observed in these experimentally induced deficiencies could be related to the requirements of manganese for the activity of enzymes that are necessary in maintenance of the skin integrity. The first group of enzymes, glycosyltranferases, functions in the synthesis of glycosaminoglycans, compounds which are components of the mucopolysaccharides of collagen in the skin as well as other tissue, etc." Good stuff, huh? She obviously uses zinc supplements.

The experiments the lady was talking about were conducted with seven men over a period of 39 days. In that same study with seven men, she found increased calcium and phosphorus in the blood along with decreased total cholesterol. From this seven-man study, it was concluded that manganese is involved in keeping skin healthy, controlling cholesterol synthesis and preventing loss of calcium from the bones. Nobody questioned the results of the small study because the researcher was a registered dietician, R.D. (she'd registered at a hotel where a dieticians' convention was held) and had later earned a doctorate in biochemistry so she had a lot of initials behind her name.

Manganese is part of an antioxidant enzyme and that may be one of its most important functions. It has also been implicated in disc and cartilage problems, glucose intolerance, reduced brain function, middle-ear imbalances, birth defects, growth retardation and PMS. There hasn't been a lot of research done with manganese but a lack of it has been blamed for a lot of medical malfeasance.

Sorry, I screwed up again. Dr. Carl Scheele, not Carol, discovered manganese, but the other stuff is right. Come to think of it, I really screwed up because the Swedes (did I tell you he was Swedish?) use Karl not Carl and Karl Scheele discovered a bunch of elements—my apologies to his descendants. I went to school in Wyoming with a girl named Karla.

Boron

Boron (B, not Bo) is named boron because, until recently, it was boring. Boron's prior claim to fame was having been part of the long-running T.V. program, "Death Valley Days," sponsored by Twenty Mule Team Borax and once hosted by Ronald Reagan before he became Governor of California. The name boron comes from…can you guess? Wrong!!! It comes from an Arabic (yes, Arabic) term meaning borax. Boron became interesting after some scientists at the USDA laboratory in Grand Forks, North Dakota (Grand Forks is west of East Grand Forks which is across the Red River in Minnesota) said boron (B) is needed in the body. The scientists at the lab across the river from East Grand Forks produced evidence that boron may play an important role in preventing osteoporosis. Results from that same lab also showed that folks who don't get enough boron can't play computer games very well.

Iodine

Iodine (I) isn't a mineral because it's a halogen, which probably doesn't mean anything to you but you've probably heard of halogen lamps and they contain iodine but not the kind used by the body. Those studying nutrition science get to study about iodine because it is needed in the body to make the thyroid hormone work properly. Iodine has a very interesting history but I'm sure students of nutrition never get to hear about it. Not so with my readers.

The fact that iodine is needed in the body was first discovered by the Chinese a long, long time ago but they didn't know it. The Chinese would eat seaweed or burnt sponge to cure big lumps in the throat. Nobody knew what to call these lumps until the French borrowed the word *gutturn* from the Latin and turned it into *goitre,* which we call goiter. Also, the references I referred to, referred to burnt sponge as the medicinal. Mr. Webster indicates that we could also say burned sponge because they've both had a match set to them. When some ancient Greek physicians (they weren't ancient then but they are now) heard about the sparked sponge treatment, they started giving burnt sponge to their patients afflicted with goiter. The remedy was very effective and, as you might expect, several Greek physicians took credit for this amazing discovery. Hippocrates, however, ended up getting all the credit because he knew about zinc and lecithin and boron and he took an oath.

Nobody knew or really cared about why sponge could cure goiter, which wasn't called goiter until the French borrowed the word *guttern* from the Latin and turned it into *goitre* which we call goiter, for a long time. Folks just chewed seaweed or chomped sponge until a

French chemist discovered iodine in seaweed just a few years before a Scandinavian chemist discovered it in sponge. These discoveries prompted a French physician to start using iodine salts to treat goiter. Back then—a lot like today—most physicians didn't care diddly-squat about learning why a disease occurred so that it could be prevented, they were just happy to have a drug treatment.

The iodine treatments didn't however go completely unnoticed. A French botanist named Chatin spent (some say wasted) 25 years of his life studying air, water, soil and food to determine how much iodine was present. He then compared his results with goiter statistics and announced to the world that iodine deficiency is the cause of goiter. Chatin went so far as to suggest that iodine be added to water supplies where the element was low. Unfortunately for the field of medicine, somebody started a rumor that Monsieur Chatin drank soymilk, like monks, to curb his sexual desires. Way back then folks knew that soymilk contains phytate which inhibits zinc absorption so they thought he was a couple pickles short of a barrel and paid no attention to him.

Luckily, a German chemist showed that iodine is a normal constituent of the body, especially the thyroid gland (amazing as it seems, this German wasn't trying to prevent or cure thyroid problems in rats. However, some Americans recently discovered that broccoli can prevent and cure ulcers in mice). Soon after scientists began to appreciate the importance of iodine, an American chemist isolated the hormone thyroxin from the thyroid gland and showed that it contained 65% iodine. The medical world finally understood why iodine is so important and wondered why somebody hadn't discovered it long before.

In case you were wondering, the word iodine comes from the Greek word *iodes* which is the color of the fumes omitted by burning iodine. Back when 'ol Hippocrates was burning sponge to produce burnt sponge, he said that when they finally discovered iodine in those sponges it should be named for the Greek word for the color produced when sponges are burned.

Iron

Iron (Fe—you were expecting Ir or Io or In, I'll bet) was discovered by some caveman who picked up a meteor (it probably wasn't a cavewoman because back in those days they were made to stay at home in the cave and do the washing, ironing and cooking). We know iron dates back to prehistoric times because writings have been found describing "the metal from heaven," a reference to the iron in meteors. More than a thousand years before Christ chased the money changers out of the Temple (now we have the CEO's of major corporations so nothing changes), iron was being obtained from ores. This ushered in the Iron Age, which women loathed until the advent of wrinkle free clothing. The chemical symbol, Fe, for iron comes from the Latin word *ferrum* for silvery solid. The Anglo-Saxons called it iron but since the Romans made such good use of it, and because there were already a bunch of I's in the symbol catalog, scientists decide to use Fe.

Iron is hooked onto some enzymes and helps them do their thing by gobbling up and spitting out electrons, but its most important job is in the protein called hemoglobin, which carries oxygen from the lungs to the cells. Without iron, hemoglobin cannot function. In fact, it can't even be produced!

Because we cannot live unless oxygen is delivered to our cells, iron is a very, very important mineral. Since iron is so important, nutrition professionals fussed and worried for years because most people, particularly women, don't get enough iron from their diets. Experts lectured about the kinds of food folks should eat to get their daily iron quota and some even went so far as to suggest supplements (sacrilege).

Then along came the late 80s when some scientists began worrying that iron might be a cause of heart disease. Within a short period of time, professionals stopped talking about iron, multivitamin supplements no longer contained iron and there were no more advertisements touting the vim and vigor restoration properties of iron supplements. Ironically, iron, one of the most important minerals in the body, suddenly became verboten just because some researcher said it might cause cholesterol to rust (those are not the terms he used but mine are simpler and mean the same thing). The rusty cholesterol guy even went so far as to suggest phlebotomy (remember that from back in the Dark Ages?) to ward off heart disease. Of course he was referring to donating blood occasionally.

Before leaving iron, I want to share with you some tidbits from an advertisement for Aphanizomenon Flos-Aquae a.k.a. Blue Green Algae. (Is that an oxymoron or is the algae blue-green?) According to the info ad I read, this stuff is the "nearly perfect food." Loaded with all kinds of nutrients, the funny colored algae is guaranteed to cure all sorts of ailments including anemia, which is caused by a lack of iron in the diet. Algae contain a lot of chlorophyll and hemoglobin is nearly identical to chlorophyll except chlorophyll contains magnesium instead of iron. The ad tells us a researcher way back in 1936 conducted a classic study in which he found that anemic patients increased hemoglobin levels faster when chlorophyll was taken with iron. This, of course, is intended to make us believe if we eat some of these algae biscuits, the chlorophyll will rush into our blood streams where iron will displace the magnesium and the chlorophyll turned hemoglobin will rush to the lungs to pick up a load of oxygen. This will most likely not happen and it sure won't unless you buy the very best variety of algae—that being stuff grown in Klamath Lake in southern Oregon.

Colloidal Myths

No section on minerals would be complete without a discussion of the infamous colloidal minerals.

Back in the roaring '20s, a sickly rancher was stumbling around in the wilds of Utah when he encountered a Paiute Indian called Chief Soaring Eagle. The chief told the rancher about a stream that had healing powers. The rancher found the stream and followed it back to its source where he found some interesting shales. The rancher made a tonic from the shales, cured himself and others, formed a company, sold the tonic and a minor legend was born. Interestingly, present-day Paiutes claim they have no knowledge of either Chief Soaring Eagle or the legendary healing powers of their ancestral waters.

When a veterinarian who likes to dress up in patriotic shirts heard about the legend, he headed for Utah and struck up a business relationship with the company started by the rancher. Then he went back home where he made an audiotape called "Dead Doctors Don't Lie!" He tells us that dead doctors don't lie because they're dead and they're dead because they failed to take daily doses of this colloidal mineral concoction which is produced from shale found only in a particular region of Utah. He made a lot of other unfounded claims prompting the rancher's company to severe ties with the vet. After the split, the animal doctor found another spot to dig up shale, formed his own company and allowed as if shale from other regions might have equally good healing powers.

Despite the hype generated by the purveyors of colloidal minerals, there is absolutely no scientific evidence demonstrating their effectiveness and certainly nothing to warrant classifying colloidals as extraordinary forms of minerals. The folks who distribute colloidal minerals claim they possess all sorts of healing powers because the product contains 75 "minerals." Actually they mean elements but we'll forgive them because most probably don't know the difference between a periodic chart and a bowling score sheet. Included in the 75 "minerals" the colloidal vendors brag about are cadmium, lead and mercury. A survey of the scientific literature shows that people who ingest cadmium, lead or mercury often exhibit peculiar behavior before succumbing to their toxic effects. Hmmm.

Antioxidants

This section is dedicated to Dr. Denham Harmon who first brought free radicals to the attention of the medical profession. He, like so many pioneers before him, was ignored and scorned for several years until science finally discovered the truth.

Some vitamins are antioxidants, some minerals are antioxidants and some things that are neither vitamins nor minerals are antioxidants so I put this section here. Years ago, prospective young Ists didn't learn much about antioxidants because nobody knew much about them. And then along came a couple of scientists who discovered a copper-containing enzyme in our bodies and wondered what the heck it did. They found out. It destroyed chemicals that could hurt cells. This made other scientists wonder about the stuff that was being destroyed and a whole new area of research was launched—the study of free radicals.

Radical thoughts

Chemists call any substance that has an odd number of electrons a radical. Most radicals quickly join up with some other radicals to form a substance that has an even number of electrons (you know, two odds make an even). Not so with the miscreants known as free radicals. They steal an electron from some unsuspecting compound and then go on their way. That's why they're called free radicals. When a free radical purloins an electron, entire cells get destroyed.

Unfortunately, free radicals are everywhere. We breath them in, we get them through our food and, as if that isn't enough, our cells manage to make a whole bunch. That's right, our cells actually make stuff that can kill them. First, the little generators called mitochondria produce the power to make cells operate, run on fuel. When that fuel is burned, exhaust is omitted and the exhaust fumes cause problems for the cells. Also, when our immune systems are at war with some invading organism, they make their own special kind of free radicals and use them for artillery. After one of these battles there are a lot of undetonated radicals scattered around, which can be disastrous for innocent cells.

Students studying to become Ists must learn and understand what free radicals do inside the body: 1. Lipid peroxidation, in which free radicals initiate damage to fat compounds in the body, causing them to turn rancid and release more free radicals; 2. Cross-linking, in which free radical reactions cause proteins and/or DNA molecules to fuse together; 3. Membrane damage, in which free radical reactions destroy the integrity of the cell membrane, which in turn interferes with the cell's ability to take in nutrients and expel wastes; 4. Lysosome damage, in which free radical reactions rupture lysosome (cell digestive particle) membranes which then spill into the cell and digest critical cell compounds; 5. Accumulation of the age pigment (lipofuscin), which may interfere with cell chemistry. It's at this point in their training that many would be Ists decide to drop out and become interior decorators, personal trainers or writers of nutrition columns.

So what happens when radicals turn fat rancid, weld DNAs together, poke holes in membranes or force cells to start collecting dye? In 1986, Dr. Jeffrey Bland listed the known disorders associated with free radicals as: adverse drug reactions, alcohol-induced liver damage, arthritic tissue damage, cancer, cardiac toxicity, cataracts, coronary heart disease, diabetic cataracts, immune hypersensitivity, inflammatory bowel disorders, neurological degeneration, red blood cell damage and traumatic inflammation. Since that time the list has grown to include impotence, hearing loss, asthma, headaches,

Alzheimer's disease, periodontal disease, ulcers, hay fever, strokes, a few I've probably missed, and hemorrhoids. (Why are they called hemorrhoids instead of asstoroids?)

With cell-generated exhaust fumes polluting our insides and the spoils of war strewn about, our cells need some protection. When our species was evolving Ma Nature decided living things should be able to make substances to protect themselves from the ravages of free radicals. That was a benevolent and protective gesture but apparently Mom didn't foresee a time when we would be threatened by herbicides, pesticides, radiation, air pollution, automobile exhaust, tobacco smoke, toxic waste, medications, exercise, stress and politicians. Things were a lot simpler in days of yore and the protection Nature provided just won't cut it in today's world. Our cells need a lot of help from the outside in order to survive the destructive forces of free radicals.

Radical Routers

The substances that destroy free radicals whether they are made inside or come from food or supplements are called antioxidants. Why, you're wondering, aren't they called antifreeradicals or simply antiradicals? What's wrong with radical routers? Let me expatiate. When I once said that to my mother, she threatened to wash my mouth out with soap. After I explained what I meant she told me to wash my hands when I was finished. Free radicals do their damage by smashing into other chemicals in order to steal an electron (they're like pickpockets). When a substance loses an electron, chemists say it has been oxidized. Thus, free radicals are oxidizers or oxidants. Thus, thus, the name antioxidant.

Shortly after the study of free radicals became a legitimate enterprise, meaning scientists could get at least a little grant money to conduct experiments, there were only five substances thought to be of any real importance as antioxidants—vitamin A, beta-carotene, vitamin C, vitamin E and selenium. Not so anymore. No sooner had beta-carotene attained superstar status than alpha-carotene (ten times more effective!!!) burst on the scene. Then came lycopene (100 times more effective than vitamin E), followed by gamma-carotene (83 times more effective than vitamin E), zeaxanthin (ten times more potent than E) and lutein (weighing in at eight times the potency of vitamin E).

Other additions to the antioxidant arsenal are glutathione and coenzyme Q-10 (cells can make these two), bioflavonoids (eriodictyol, hesperitin, hesperidin, rutin, queercetin, quercetrin, citrin, narigen and esculin), bilberry, gallocatechin gallate (green tea), wine, garlic (which contains the antioxidants allicin, selenium and germanium—yes, germanium) and ginkgo biloba. Memorizing the ever-growing list of antioxidants also encourages prospective Ists to seek careers in less confusing fields.

Another antioxidant that is starting to curry favor is curcumin, which is found in curry spices. Researchers think the low incidence of Alzheimer's disease in India is due to the people's consumption of spices containing the antioxidant. They believe this because mice fed curcumin don't get Alzheimer's as readily as mice fed plain, unspiced, unseasoned, just plain yucky mice food. These experiments were done by some goofy Americans as were the ones that showed old rats fed blueberries (which contain antioxidants) could beat young rats on memory tests (I'm serious).

Transcript from blueberry tests:

"Alright, Methuselah, tell me what you had for dinner ten days ago."

"Oh, Alex, that's easy. I had my usual rat cuisine garnished with generous helpings of blueberries."

"Very good. Now, Little Mikey, tell me what you had for dinner last night."

"Can I pick a different category, Alex?"

"Answer the question, Mikey."

"Well, it wasn't blueberries. Was it?"

"No."

"I just can't remember. I'm like so stressed out with these tests. What I am doing taking memory tests? I'm a rat!"

This book would have gone to press months ago but I kept holding off because I wanted you the reader to be up to date on the latest developments in the quest to keep rats and mice alive and healthy with antioxidants. Finally I said "Enough!" and put the finishing touches on it. If I have left out any antioxidants, I apologize. If the book sells well I'll include any I missed in the next edition.

Most of the really good antioxidants can be found in plants, which troubles me more than just a little. Remember I told you cells make free radicals during their everyday routine of living? And I also told you they try to make antioxidants so the radicals won't destroy them. I'm curious as to why it is that plants have to make copious quantities of really potent antioxidants. The Ists tell us to eat a lot of veggies but I'm beginning to wonder if that really is such a good idea.

Pomp and Circumstance

Finally, it's graduation day! After losing their virginity in a dingy motel in Florida over Spring Break, gaining 30 pounds from dormitory food, puking up their guts at fraternity parties, trashing a police car after learning their team didn't make the "big dance," cheating on a few exams, attending several anti-[fill in your favorite] rallies and memorizing the names of the important antioxidants, our nutrition students collect their diplomas with pride and dignity (and a lot of unpaid loans). Tassels tickling their noses, the graduates grasp their credentials knowing they have been granted a degree by a respected university after completing a thorough, scientifically sound training program.

The inspirational words of the graduation speaker have barely begun to fade from memory when our matriculates are accosted by frustrated parents wondering why they didn't enroll in one of those less expensive "universities" where you don't have to live in dorms or even attend classes. Befuddled, the legitimate Ists soon learn that wannabe "nutritionists" can easily obtain degrees and certificates without having to go through the rigors of learning about the complex carbohydrates or the lipid lexicon or who discovered what vitamin or what free radicals are or how antioxidants work. And the names of all those antioxidants—heaven forbid!

Wastrels who decide to enroll in one of the scofflaw "schools" will never have to worry about the alumni association asking for money. Nor will they ever read a report in the paper describing how their old alma mater has been put on probation for violating NCAA rules and procedures. On the other hand, they will never see a graduate from their "school" in the NBA or NFL. Neither will they have the pleasure of wearing a mum at a homecoming game or marching to the sounds of Pomp and Circumstance. What they will see is the "President" of their "university" indicted for fraud.

The "universities" I'm talking about dispense with such frivolities as sports, fraternities, sororities, classes or education. No "To the Tables Down at Mory's," "Gaudeamus Egitur," or "Fight on for Old" at these institutions. They are diploma mills, established for the sole purpose of taking your money and mailing you a degree. The more you pay, the higher the degree.

Degree mills have been around for hundreds of years, and they are still flourishing all over the world. Like drug dealers and pornographers, diploma mills stay in business because people keep buying their products. Dozens of places offer Bachelor's, Master's, Doctorates, law and medical degrees, with no questions asked. Pay the fees—anywhere from one dollar to several thousand—hang your diploma. You won't find ivy-covered halls at these "institutions." The campuses are found in dilapidated old buildings, garages, home offices and little retail establishments where they print diplomas while you wait. Transcripts are also available (cum laude comes at a higher price).

Tuition at the diploma mills is not a problem. At a "university" in California (which I can proudly say was kicked out of Nevada), one can enroll in a "Nutritionist" course for less than $100, including the cost of one "textbook." After taking two open-book tests, which anybody with the I.Q. of a squid could pass, the "school" will send a gold-sealed certificate announcing you have graduated Cum Laude.

Slackers who don't want to bother with a diploma mill can apply to a "lost diploma replacement service." A ne'er-do-well has but to simply tell one of these services they had a legitimate degree but lost it, and it will be replaced for a modest fee (fifty bucks for a Harvard "Doctor of Neurosurgery" diploma). For students actually enrolled at legitimate institutions of higher learning, but who are too lazy to put forth the effort, there are term paper and dissertation writing services. Several distribute catalogs listing thousands of already-written term papers they will sell. If a topic isn't listed in their catalog, they will gladly write anything from a short paper to a major dissertation for $7 to $10 a page.

Ists That Ain't

The eager Ists have barely shed the depression of degree mills when they learn with dismay that anyone who so chooses may designate herself/himself a "nutritionist." All that is required is the ability to read and report or distort the results of experiments conducted by competent scientists.

One of the most infamous self-styled "nutritionists" actually earned a degree at a reputable institution. In the spring of 1931, Harold Frederick Caplan graduated from the University of Alabama (The Crimson Tide, "Bear" Bryant) with a major in English and a minor in political science. Despite having virtually no nutrition or health science training—two hours of physiology and eight hours of elementary chemistry—Carlton Fredericks (1910-1987), the name he later adopted, was hired by the U.S. Vitamin Corporation to write advertising copy and give sales talks. While performing these duties he adopted the title of "nutrition educator."

Soon after taking the position with USVC, records of the Magistrates' Court of New York City show that Fredericks began diagnosing patients as well as prescribing vitamins for their illnesses. Following an investigation by the New York State Department of Education, he was charged with unlawful practice of medicine. He pleaded guilty, paid a fine of $500 (rather than spend three months in jail) and joined the rolls of those with criminal convictions in connection with nutrition frauds.

Fredericks enrolled in New York University's School of Education and received a master's degree in 1949, and a night-school Ph.D. in communications in 1955. The title of his doctoral thesis was "A Study of the Responses of a Group of Adult Female Listeners to a Series of

Educational Radio Programs." These were his own radio programs, broadcast on New York City's WOR and distributed at times to other stations. Fredericks' thesis analyzed how much of certain things he said on his program were retained by its listeners and how it affected their food-buying habits.

Although Fredericks was never enrolled in a nutrition course he used his doctorate in communications to his advantage. He was introduced as "Dr. Fredericks" on radio and television programs and, since he was dispensing medical advice, listeners assumed he was a medical doctor.

During a court case in 1965, Dr. Victor Herbert, called as an expert witness, described Fredericks as a "charlatan." The defense objected but was overruled after Dr. Herbert read aloud the Random House Dictionary definition of charlatan: "one who pretends to have more knowledge than he possesses; quack."

Until his death, Fredericks considered himself an expert and gave self-diagnosis and self-treatment advice in books and in articles for health-food publications. The covers of some of his books describe him as "America's Foremost Nutritionist." Toward the end of his career, "Dr. Fredericks" conducted "nutrition consultations" for $200 each at the offices of Dr. Robert Atkins. A heavy smoker, he died of a heart attack at the age of 76.

A long list

The nutrition industry is a lot of legerdemain (a.k.a. smoke and mirrors). I originally intended to mention the names of several scalawags involved in dubious healthcare schemes and sporting questionable credentials but decided against it in order to keep this book from becoming too voluminous. While searching the literature and the Internet, I discovered that the list of charlatans connected with nutrition is long and formidable and it was impossible to determine just who should be included and who should be overlooked. I devised a rating scale, one misdeed being the least dishonest and ten the most, but this didn't cull the list much so I limited the discussion to "Dr. Fredericks" to remind you that there are many Ists who ain't. Scouring through the writings, schemes and antics of some of these people I realized that the title of this book is really a double entendre since "funny" refers to more than just humorous.

In the process of researching cheaters, I came across a website called Quackwatch, which lambastes several "notorious" individuals (Linus Pauling was one). After reading the records of many of these people I was surprised my name was not included on the list. Many of the outlaws on the Quackwatch list are guilty of no more than encouraging the use of food supplements and/or specific foods to ward off disease.

Section Two:

BEING AN IST

Things Ists Do and Argue About

The Nutrition Expert

After they stop studying nutrition, graduate and become Ists, our experts join the ranks of those who come up with clever statements like, "You are what you eat." (This may have been stolen. See appendix 3.) Gems like this let us know in no uncertain terms if you eat fat, you're fat. Eat tomatoes, you're a tomato. Eat fruits, you're a fruit. Eat convenience foods, you're fast, cheap and easy. Eat a balanced diet and you become a scale.

These talented punsters also gave us "empty Calories." This would be the opposite of full (burp) Calories.

"The whiter the bread, the sooner you're dead," tells us we should eat toast.

Some students do graduate work to earn an M.S. degree (not to be confused with Ms.) and learn more pithy platitudes like, "Americans have the most expensive urine in the world." That may be so but Prostate's Pee Shop has great pre-holiday sales and they take American Express.

Really motivated students continue graduate work until they obtain a whole bunch of letters behind their name: B.S., M.S., Ph.D., B.F.D., B.V.D, C.D., C.D.ROM, I.D., L.D., O.D., R.D., V.D.

Many graduates in nutritional science go on to become county extension agents, teachers and dieticians. If they sign a book at the hotel where a dieticians' convention is being held, they become a registered dietician (R.D.) and if they eat too much they become an L.D. (large dietician).

County extension agents have the most fun and perform the greatest service because they answer—often in papers or over radio and television—important questions about food.

Question: "Do I need to cut my turkey's head off before I poke it in the oven?"

"No. It's best if you don't because so many folks get blood on the carcass and that's not healthy. Be sure you pluck the bird though because feathers are flammable. Also, be sure to wash the feet and legs because those birds walk around in that nasty old poop all day."

Question: "Where can I get salmonella?"

"Oh, I'm so happy you asked because I encourage you to get all the salmonella you can. Salmonella is a female fish that comes from the Northwest. It contains omega-3 fatty acids that are good for your cardiovascular system. We nutritionists just love to use big scientific words. Just go to your local market and find the fish section. Since the population is mostly female, you'll get plenty of salmonella."

Question: "Joe Bob caught some fish in the pond down by the thermometer plant. He said they ooze out these tiny shiny drops. I think it's mercury, what do you think?"

"Oh, my. Those are fish eggs. Society folks call them caviar. Tell Joe Bob to put them in a cup beside some crackers and serve them at his next Super Bowl party. His friends will think they're to die for."

Those who teach nutrition convince their students to ignore any so called advances in nutrition knowledge and stay with the tried and true. "If it ain't broke, don't fix it. Everything we need to know about nutrition was discovered before or right after World War II. Do not, I repeat, do not listen to anybody who tries to tell you the RDAs are inadequate. People have lived and died with them for years."

Expert Ists often sit around reading and criticizing the work of scientists who question the adequacy of our everyday diets and dare to suggest food supplements may help us live healthier longer. Skilled, shrewd dieticians offer non-sequitors like, "You get what you need with your knife and fork." When that was first ridiculed, they added a spoon. Another favorite of dieticians is, "More research is needed."

After the 37th study involving hundreds of volunteers showed that children grow better when fed, several dieticians, when asked to comment, responded with, "There isn't enough data for a proper evaluation. More research is needed."

The Great Food Pyramids

Armed with their degrees and initials, experts who obtain employment with the U.S. Department of Agriculture find themselves building pyramids. The structures built by the skilled professionals are called the great Food Guide Pyramids and they're definitely not listed in the Wonders of the World. These look like the ancient Egyptian pyramids but have chambers filled with bread, fish, chicken, fruits and vegetables instead of gold, silver, fine linens and decaying mummies. The USDA built the food pyramids, and, because opinions about what's healthy and what's not have changed over the years, the agency has several pyramids on their property in Beltsville, Maryland. You won't find pictures of food pyramids in geography books but there are some nice photos in nutrition texts.

If you regularly read the hieroglyphics on a food pyramid, you can avoid dietary sloth and always be healthy. The lower chamber of the food pyramid is chock full of bread, cereal, rice and pasta with instructions on how to eat these. There are two chambers above the lower, one filled with fruit, the other with vegetables. The walls of the second story chamber contain no recipes because they want you to eat these foods fresh. Some wag did, however, scratch a note on the wall of one of the chambers reading, "The FDA sucks." Ascending the pyramid you find two more chambers, one containing meat, poultry, fish, beans, eggs and nuts; the other milk, yogurt and cheese. The meat and poultry chamber cautions us about undercooking. The top chamber—the "Forbidden" chamber—contains fats, oils and sweets. A sign on the upper chamber door reads, "Use Sparingly."

Hell no, we won't C H O

The last stone had barely been put in place on the latest Beltsville pyramid when protestors, mostly supporters of Drs. Atkins and Sears, began gathering at the base of the structure. The lower chamber of the food pyramid, filled with bread, cereal, rice and pasta, has too much carbohydrate according to the agitators. Equally bad, the chamber archives don't distinguish between processed white bread and fiber-rich whole grain. Well, excuse me!

Dr. Arthur Agatston, director of the Cardiac Prevention Center at Mount Sinai Hospital in Miami Beach, FL says, "Think of white bread as consuming alcohol on an empty stomach. Whole grain is consuming alcohol on a full stomach. If you take alcohol on an empty stomach, the alcohol is quickly absorbed into your bloodstream and you get drunk. You can get drunk on sugar, too."

Fraternity man: "Remember, don't eat anything after noon."

Other frat. man: "Why?"

Fraternity man: "We're serving white bread at the party tonight."

Other frat. man: "Whoa! Sounds like a blast."

The chanting demonstrators at the base of the pyramid feel the bottom chamber should be filled with all the fat stuff while the carbohydrates are relegated to the upper, forbidden, chamber. According to Dr. Robert Atkins, "Fat satiates the appetite. Fat stops carbohydrate craving. And fat, in the absence of carbohydrates, accelerates the burning of stored fat." The placard-toting activists might believe their esteemed guru but hundreds, maybe thousands, of professionals who claim low-carb diets are unhealthy would like to see Dr. Atkins wrapped like a mummy and entombed in one of the pyramids.

Eldermids

The employees of the USDA laboratory in Grand Forks North Dakota haven't completed a pyramid as of this writing (they're probably waiting for the snow to melt) but the folks at the Human Nutrition Research Center on Aging at Tufts University in Boston have. The Boston professionals decided to construct a pyramid especially for "70-plus adults." This pyramid is equipped with elevators, is wheel chair accessible on each level and is designed for the chronologically challenged. Because older people eat less, the Boston pyramid is narrower than those in Beltsville which were designed for the young and spry. State of the art water fountains have been installed on each level to remind geezers to drink at least eight glasses of water a day. This addition was one of the most controversial because some professionals were concerned the pyramid would flood. Others worried the seniors might drink too much water and spoil their appetites or worse, become incontinent (the pyramid isn't equipped with bathrooms).

The Boston pyramid is truly modern and innovative throughout (knowing elderly citizens like an evening cocktail, one of the designers of this pyramid suggested selling alcohol on the top level but she was overruled and the hooch was left out completely). In addition to hieroglyphics recommending fewer servings of foodstuff from each level, this progressive structure is topped with a flag. The banner reads "Use vitamin supplements." Can you believe it? Nutrition professionals recommending supplements! Before long even the pyramids at Beltsville might be sporting streamers heralding the value of daily vitamin/mineral supplements.

They're everywhere

First Egypt and now the world. Pyramids have cropped up everywhere. Disenchanted with the shabby construction of the Great USDA Food Pyramid, dissenters throughout the world began enslaving dieticians and constructing their own. We now have the Healthy Eating Pyramid, the California Cuisine Pyramid, the Mediterranean Diet Pyramid (more about this later), the Soul Food Pyramid and the Walter Willett Food Pyramid.

Each pyramid is—as you probably imagined—shaped like the pyramids of old but the contents of the chambers within vary markedly. The Soul Food structure is very colorful. It's our only ethnic food pyramid. It was designed and built to educate individuals that traditionally eat "soul food."

The California creation is filled with—as expected—fruits and nuts and twigs and sprigs. The bottom contains veggies and fruits, but not just any kind of fruits and vegetables. They must be phytonutrient-rich vegetables and fruits. Above that are high fiber grains and other vegetable groups and protein-rich food groups. The top chamber is definitely unique since it's packed with "Taste Enhancers." Exotic spices, no doubt.

The Healthy Eating Pyramid was built in Australia and a lot of beer was consumed during its construction. This structure has three levels: Eat More, Eat Moderately and Eat Small Amounts. The lower level sports vegetables, fruits, lentils, dried peas, beans, lentils, breads and cereals (preferably whole grain). The second chamber has moderate stocks of fish, lean meats, eggs, chicken (preferably without skin), and dairy products such as milk, cheese and yoghurt (their spelling). The top includes fats, oils (butter and margarine) and sugar. Listen up, mate. "The foods at the top of the pyramid should be restricted because they provide many kilojoules without providing much in the way of nutrients."

Dr. Walter Willett, chairman of the department of nutrition at Harvard, designed and single handedly built a pyramid which has two "Use Sparingly" top chambers. One contains red meat and butter; the other is packed with white rice, white bread, potatoes, pasta and sweets. The Atkins and Sears supporters have tried on numerous occasions to destroy Willett's pyramid but the attempts were unsuccessful because the structure is just too sound. It is firmly attached to a foundation made of Daily Exercise and Weight Control.

The food pyramids are supposed to remind you to eat a variety of foods every day. Because there are so many scattered across our great nation and throughout the world, the next time you're on vacation you might spot one in the distance. Take a snapshot, enlarge it and hang it in the kitchen for all to admire.

Food Labels

Another very important topic our nutrition specialists deal with is food labels. Many years ago families sat at the breakfast table and conversed with each other about their plans for the day while Dad read the newspaper and grunted approval. Then somebody in the government decided children and adults should read more. At about the same time, another government employee thought we should have labels on our food products so folks would know just exactly what they're eating. This was so people would know what to expect when they looked in the mirror after eating a meal. Never wasteful and always involved in education, government officials decided to combine two programs, reading and labeling. The contemporary breakfast table—if the family even bothers—is surrounded by children and Moms digesting (no pun intended) the valuable information on milk cartons and cereal boxes while Dad reads the paper. The kids go off to school to learn more reading skills, leaving Mom and Dad to further improve their reading skills at work or by perusing food labels on canned or packaged goods and frozen dinners.

Early food labels were, for the most part, ignored. In addition to serving size, the label told how many servings in a container. For example, serving size = one peanut; servings per container = 429. The label told us how many Calories (more about this later) were in a serving along with how many grams of protein, carbohydrate and fat. This, of course, meant nothing to the anxious reader who wanted to know if the heroine swallowed the fish whole because (1) we don't use the metric system so nobody knew what the hell a gram was and (2) very few readers, with the exception of those who were employed as Ists, knew how many Calories were in fats, carbohydrates and protein. The old labels listed protein as well as the vitamins and minerals found in the food and told us what percentage of the U.S. RDA (U. S. Recommended Daily Allowance) of each was in a serving.

A very confusing sidebar

By definition, Recommended Dietary Allowances (RDAs) are "the levels of intake of essential nutrients that, on the basis of scientific knowledge, are judged by the Food and Nutrition Board to be adequate to meet the known nutrient needs of practically all healthy persons." Do you feel all warm and fuzzy? The Food and Nutrition Board (experts who help create confusion) state that "the RDAs should not be confused with U.S. Recommended Daily Allowances (U.S.RDAs)—a set of values derived from the 1968 RDAs by the Food and Drug Administration—a subsidiary of Monsanto Chemical—as standards for nutritional labeling." Well, of course, the FNBRDAs shouldn't be confused with the FDARDAs. I'm not confused. Are you? Why didn't the FDA make some recommendations and call them the EATs (Eat All This)?

I digressed. The RDAs, not to be confused with the U.S.RDAs, came into existence in the 1940s and have been the subject of criticism since. For example, in 1986 the National Academy of Sciences rejected the minor changes recommended in the RDAs, stating: "...the RDAs should be more than just the avoidance of nutritional deficiency diseases." I'm not certain what was meant by that statement but criticism from the National Academy is not to be taken lightly.

From the National Institute on Aging: "RDAs should be seriously reconsidered as it relates to nutrient need of the older, aged segment of our population to help promote disease resistance." This was especially biting criticism considering the fact most of the Food and Nutrition Board members are a week older than dirt.

The RDAs were and still are designed to "prevent deficiency

diseases in most healthy people." While the goal might be noble, attainment of the goal leaves much to be desired. The deficiency diseases the RDAs are designed to prevent—scurvy, pellagra, beriberi—faded into oblivion decades ago.

Excitement on your packages

Back to labeling. Disgruntled by the lack of information on the early labels, the RDAs and the score of the Dallas Cowboys vs. the Washington Redskins game, an ambitious employee of the Food and Drug Association (FDA a.k.a. the Faster Death Alliance) marched into the office of the director and whined, "I think our agency is being shortchanged because of those people who work in the barns out there in Beltsville."

"Why is that?" the director inquired.

"The USDA is supposed to be involved with cotton and cows, not food. They've enslaved their employees to build food pyramids, they put out booklets with clever titles like 'You Are What You Eat' and some of their employees have done some good research with food."

"Yes, that's true."

"Our agency has food in its name but theirs doesn't. It's time we did something with food other than just trying to ban food supplements."

The director thought a moment and with unprecedented speed the FDA entered the food fray. The director called the boss at the USDA and suggested the two agencies work together (nudge, nudge, wink, wink) to compile an understandable set of dietary guidelines.

Soon, new, improved dietary guidelines were issued (by the FDA) and put into law. The new guidelines included Recommended Daily Intakes (RDIs) to replace the RDAs. The differences were slight but showed the FDA was flexing its muscles. Food labeling was completely revamped with the intent of giving us simpler and much more complete information.

While the serving size in grams (even the FDA ignored the fact we're not a metric society) and number of servings remained, the numbers telling us how much we're getting were changed to percent daily values. Rather than simply telling us what percentage of the new and improved RDI we're getting, the new labels show what percentage we get by eating either a 2000 Calorie per day diet or a 2500 Calorie per day diet. Thus, the RDIs are expressed as %DVs. Unfortunately, there are no instructions explaining how one determines if they are eating 2000 Calories per day or 40,000 Calories per day. This new label is so much simpler.

For those totally bored out of their gourd, the new food labels offer a quick course on the nutritional value of a food product. Toting some well known, everyday facts (i.e. 1 gram fat = 9 Calories; 1 gram protein = 4 Calories; 1 gram carbohydrate = 4 Calories; 1 gram alcohol = 7 Calories; 1 gram diet Coke = 0 Calories), the extremely gifted consumer can quickly glean important information such as: How many Calories would you get from fat, if you ate one serving of the food item? How many Calories would you consume, if you ate the entire contents of this food item? (Pig!) Assuming you followed a 2000 kcal diet, what is the recommended amount of cholesterol per day? If you ate one portion of this food item, how many milligrams (mg) of cholesterol would you have consumed? Assuming that you followed a 2500 kcal diet, what is the recommended daily intake of fiber? If you ate two portions of this food item, how many grams of fiber would you consume? (Don't even think about eating three portions.) What percentage (%) of the daily value is this? What % of the total fat is saturated fat? How many Calories do you get from each gram of carbohydrate? How many legs on a centipede? How many carbohydrate Calories do you get per serving of this food item? What is the recommended daily intake of sodium for someone consuming a 2000 kcal diet? Who killed J.R.? How many mg of sodium do you get from three servings of this food item? What is the % of Daily Value if you consume three servings? (You've already had too much sodium, forget the three servings.) How many portions would you need to consume to exceed the recommended daily amount of sodium? Assume that you are following a 2000 kcal diet. When looking at this Nutrition Facts Label, does a serving of this food provide more fat, carbohydrates or protein grams? Would you consider this pre-cardiac arrest cuisine? What can you say about this food in regards to its vitamin A content? Would you say that it's a good or poor source of vitamin A? Are rabbits or carrots a better source of vitamin A? What is the total volume of this food package? What is the total volume of your butt? If there are three grams of protein per serving, how many calories of protein is that? All this and more from the food label on a miniature candy bar.

For one with a Ph.D. in Nutritional Science and a few years post-doctoral education, the new, improved labels might be more informative and complete. The average person would find the introduction to a textbook on advanced calculus more helpful.

The FDA is lobbying vigorously to have labels put on all food products. I'm wondering if they'll want individual labels on each grape or pea or if the person at the checkout counter will have to thumb through a packet full of labels until they find the right one to poke in the bag along with your green beans. Imagine the scene at the doughnut counter: You've picked up your coffee in one hand and with other you're about to take a bite out of that golden, glazed gob of goodness when the clerk tacks a nutrition label onto your morning indulgence. Consider beer, liquor and wine containers. After the Surgeon General warns us against having a baby or driving a tractor while drinking this brew, the FDA will lecture us about swilling "empty Calories."

If government agencies keep improving labeling information, booklets containing vital information about which Greek word the name of the product was derived from, how many jobs developed because of the product, how many jobs were lost when the labeling company moved to Mexico, how many worms were run over when the product was harvested, who killed J. R., the age and marital status of the farmer's daughter, who to contact if the product spoils because your freezer stopped running after the neighbor's kid pulled the plug, will one day be attached to every food product.

Cholesterol,
The Cuddly Puppy of the Health Profession

Heart disease is one of the leading causes of death in the world today but the cause of this malady remains a mystery. To make up for their inadequacy the Ists in the health profession have found a scapegoat—cholesterol.

Cholesterol is a fat and all the hype surrounding it is a big fat lie. To begin with, health professionals tell folks there are two kinds of cholesterol, LDL (Lethal Damn Lipids) and HDL (Healthy Decent Lipids). The average Joe and Joette are led to believe their blood is a battlefield where the evil, bad cholesterol (LDL) and the healthy, good cholesterol (HDL) wage constant war against each other.

Ask any fat chemist or thin chemist or lipid chemist how many kinds of cholesterol there are and they will look at you like you're speaking Klingon and just upchucked a hairball. There is one cholesterol, technically known as cyclopentanoperhydrophenanthrene (look who's talking Klingon now). Because cholesterol is a fat, it cannot, I repeat, cannot move through the blood by itself. Cholesterol needs something to transport it from the liver to the cells where it's needed. A protein transporter made in the liver, by Liver Union employees, does that job. The protein is called the low-density lipoprotein or LDL. When cells are ready to trade in their old, used cholesterol for a new (not improved, just new) model, it must be transported back to the liver where it is dismantled and used for parts. The high-density lipoprotein or HDL provides transportation from the cells back to the liver. Thus, there are two kinds of proteins that move cholesterol, not two different kinds of cholesterol.

When physicians examine the organs of people who have had a heart attack, they often find clogged arteries leading from the heart. The vessels are clogged because they are filled with, you guessed it, cholesterol. "Well, duh," is the response of responsible, competent scientists. The arteries were somehow damaged and cholesterol is used to help repair the damage. The greater the damage, the more the material needed to repair it. Also, the cholesterol found in the predamaged vessels was brought there by that villainous low-density lipoprotein (LDL). Because heart attacks occur in vessels filled with cholesterol and because LDL brought it to the site, both have become scapegoats for a problem medical science has yet to resolve.

Consider the following analogy. During the spring, a heavy rainstorm accompanied by strong winds causes water to leak through your roof and into the house where it causes damage to floors, walls and furnishings. Hoping to prevent a reoccurrence of the devastation, you replace the roofing shingles with new ones. Later that summer, lightning strikes your house causing considerable damage. Would you blame the new shingles and the contractor who delivered and installed them for the lightning damage? Of course not.

There is no sound basis to the diet-heart-cholesterol connection contrived by the government, academia and the food and pharmaceutical industries. The hoax is maintained for and nourished by greed and profit. No scientific evidence supports claims that a reduction of dietary cholesterol will increase the life of an individual. People who have high levels of cholesterol live as long as or longer than those with low cholesterol. Including two whole eggs per day has shown no significant effect on serum cholesterol levels of normal humans. Overwhelming evidence indicates that diet has little or nothing to do with coronary heart disease.

At least 60% of people who suffer heart attacks do not have elevated blood cholesterol levels. According to a former medical director of the Framingham Cardiovascular Institute, more than one in three people have blood cholesterol levels between 150 and 200 and twice as many people with life-long cholesterol levels in this range have heart attacks as do people with cholesterol over 300! "More than half the heart attacks out there occur in people who have normal cholesterol levels, don't smoke, and have few other risk factors," commented a chief of cardiovascular medicine at Brigham and Women's Hospital in Boston.

They lowered the bar

The response to the pronouncements stating that elevated cholesterol isn't the cause of heart disease will surely renew your faith in the health profession. In 2001 an "expert panel" gathered together by the National Institutes of Health voted to lower the level of LDL-cholesterol (remember, that's the evil twin) considered to be healthy. Confronted by statistics indicating more than half of those suffering from heart disease have normal levels of cholesterol, the committee decided to change the rules for what constitutes normal. Previously, 120 metric things was said to be alright but now you can have only 100 or you'll be strapped to a gurney, wheeled off to surgery, cut open and subjected to triple by-pass.

"That'll show 'em," the chairman declared. "Now at least half of the people with heart disease will have elevated blood cholesterol."

The same committee—not to be deterred while on a roll—stated that drug treatment should be started at 130 instead of the previous 160. Either these experts aren't the brightest crayons in the box or their stock portfolios are heavily weighted in the pharmaceutical sector.

Cholesterol alone isn't a cause of heart problems. Cholesterol-lowering measures in the United States have fueled a $60 billion per year industry but have not saved the citizens from the ravages of heart disease. And that's not funny.

If not cholesterol, then what? Until medical researchers get over their fixation with cholesterol, we'll have to do what Dr. Albert Szent-

Gyorgyi did and call it "Godnose." Maybe—probably—there are several Godnoses. If cholesterol did spontaneously build up by itself and form plaque, all our capillaries would quickly plug and we'd all die in a matter of hours. Arterial walls normally are very slick—like a non-stick coating. However, after a tear, scuff or chemical injury on the inner arterial wall, a cholesterol "scab" can form. This is similar to the scab that forms when you cut your skin—except it happens on the inside, and the way it happens is somewhat different.

Plaque buildup occurs as part of the protective healing process (and all along you thought it was because you didn't brush your teeth). The arterial plaque is composed of fifteen or so different materials including cholesterol, triglycerides, phospholipids, etc. Plaque formation starts immediately after artery walls have been attacked by substances that are toxic to the wall. Some current suspects are an enzyme called xanthine oxidase and the hormone insulin. Antioxidants help control xanthine oxidase while exercise, chromium picolinate and moderate carbohydrate consumption keep insulin in check. If one or both of these suspects are indicted, drugs to lower cholesterol could become a part of medical history.

More hoaxes on the horizon?

Because of the fixation with cholesterol, there has been an explosive growth of industries making incredible profits based on cholesterol measurement, low-cholesterol foods and cholesterol-reducing drugs. However, information from carefully conducted studies keeps coming in and the cholesterolophiles may one day have to give up their sacred cardiovascular disease icon. Unfortunately, there may be some other cons along the way.

The nutrition establishment is slowly coming around to the indisputable fact that cholesterol itself doesn't cause cardiovascular problems. The American College of Physicians (banned by the NCAA from all athletic competition for recruiting students who already graduated) stated in 1996 that regular cholesterol testing isn't necessary for everyone. According to its new guidelines, men under age 35, women under age 45, or persons over 75 don't need a test unless they smoke or have a family history of heart disease, high blood pressure, or diabetes. For healthy men 35 to 65 and women 45 to 65, testing is "appropriate but not mandatory." The group finds "there's little evidence that lowering cholesterol in such individuals helps prevent illness or death."

As the demise of cholesterol looms, the pharmaceutical gurus seek other profit producers and may have found what they're seeking in viruses, *chlamydia pneumonia* being one. An article in *Newsweek* (August 11, 1997) states that, "whatever their age, sex, or nationality, people with sclerotic arteries tend to show signs of infection. They say this bug (*C. pneumonia*) never shows up in otherwise healthy tissue."

A subsequent, more in-depth article appeared in the November/ December issue of *Health* magazine. The article starts by admitting that cholesterol is not the sole cause of heart attacks because high cholesterol doesn't generate higher occurrences of real life cardiovascular disease. The article mentions a study where over half the cardiovascular victims carried antibodies to *C. pneumonia*. The study also references another study that stated: "People with and without blocked arteries were likely to have antibodies to *C. pneumonia*, but levels averaged 25 percentage points higher among the heart patients."

Although the presence of a virus in people with heart disease does not prove its guilt, another drug company bonanza may be in store. One *chlamydia* researcher stated, "I'm telling you, they are going to start putting azithromycin (an antibiotic) in the drinking water." Since drug companies spent millions of dollars developing and promoting cholesterol-lowering drugs, responsible professionals are concerned the companies may soon introduce a new wave of "preventive" antibiotic drugs. This would be a disaster because widespread use of powerful antibiotics could create drug resistance in other germs that attack the respiratory system, including *C. pneumonia* itself.

More edification

Cholesterol, due to greed and poor science, is depicted as a dangerous culprit when in fact it's a very important chemical. Cholesterol has been vilified, maligned, denigrated, belittled, disparaged, slandered, criticized and pilloried. (These are all synonyms. Is there another word for synonym?) But the fact is, our bodies simply cannot function without it. Cholesterol is so important that the body produces it in large quantities—about five times as much as you eat. That's why it's nearly impossible to lower your cholesterol level more than a small amount by giving up savory bacon and eggs and mouth-watering pizza. All cells contain it and all tissues make it. Cholesterol is so important that every cell regulates its own level internally. Cholesterol gives cell membranes their integrity and strength; without cholesterol, we'd be soft, flabby, and worm-like—about the consistency of a jellyfish hung on a skeleton (I know people who look like that and they eat a lot of cholesterol). Cholesterol helps make it possible for cells to control what comes in and what goes out.

Bone would be hollow and brittle if it weren't for cholesterol and protein. Cholesterol has a major structural role in the brain, where it's found in high concentrations. Now isn't that a kick? The very substance that professionals—who are a few shingles shy on the roof—implore us to eliminate from our bodies is needed to make the brain work. I know what you're thinking and you're right—many health professionals have low cholesterol levels and are trying to pull the rest of us down to their level. Even though the brain needs cholesterol, there are some "experts" who are trying to convince us high blood cholesterol can lead to Alzheimer's disease.

The vitamin D produced inside your body comes from cholesterol. Bile, a chemical manufactured by the liver and essential for proper fat digestion, is produced from cholesterol. If you think the story about olestra was frightening, try to imagine what life would be like if you didn't have cholesterol helping to break up fats as they pass through your intestine. Those big greasy chemical lumps would silently slip into your large intestine where water would rush in to try and float them out before they clogged the drain pipes. All that fluid would cause serious "anal leakage" a.k.a. diarrhea. According to one of my sources, four out of five people suffer from occasional diarrhea—does that mean that one enjoys it?

I could go on for several pages ranting about the benefits of cholesterol, but I won't. The following segment, from the website of The Weston A. Price Foundation, Washington, DC (www.westonaprice.org) describes the importance of cholesterol in alarming terms.

FOR IMMEDIATE RELEASE

CHOLESTEROL THEORY WIPES OUT HUMAN RACE

PLANET EARTH, April 9, 2057 - A faulty theory on the origin and cause of heart disease, introduced on Planet Earth 100 years prior to this date, has caused the demise of the human race, according to a Pleiadean delegation report. The theory led to food choices that proved lethal to humans over several generations.

"We were surprised at the rapidity of its effects," said the commission's chairman, "and the tenacity of the theory. Even when infertility and early death became widespread, humans did not question the validity of the basic assumptions."

The delegation, which visits Planet Earth once every fifty earth years on fact-finding missions, estimated the decrease in earthling numbers at almost 99 percent. Only pockets of isolated populations and some descendants of impoverished dairy farmers, too poor to purchase supermarket foods, remained.

Proponents of the cholesterol theory maintained that animal fats and cholesterol from animal foods were the cause of heart disease. Vegetable oils gradually replaced

animal fats in the human diet as Earth-dwellers sought to lower their blood cholesterol below the levels needed to produce reproductive hormones. The introduction of imitation foods rich in plant-based estrogens, and of plant sterols into commonly eaten foods, exacerbated the antifertility effects.

Humans were also encouraged to take drugs to lower cholesterol levels and these had side effects such as cancer, which contributed to the population decline. And heart disease increased, in spite of rigid adherence to cholesterol-lowering regimes. Low cholesterol levels also contributed to an increase in deaths from suicide and violence. In addition, children experienced growth problems and increasing numbers failed to reach sexual maturity. The investigators cited the lack of protective nutrients found in animal fats as a factor exacerbating all these conditions.

Ironically, a few earthling scientists had warned against the effects of diets based on vegetable oils, the commission found. But these souls were either ignored or persecuted. Over time, mental ability declined with great numbers of children experiencing learning difficulties and attention deficit disorder. Alzheimer's and senility increased among the elderly. Humans could no longer make sense of ancestral dietary traditions or of published studies on the role of animal fats in human nutrition.

The real enemy, according to the report, was fear. "Humans were taught to fear the very foods that had made their evolution possible," said the observers. "They were very gullible and believed the advertisements and pronouncements of those who profited from the sale of vegetable oils and cholesterol-lowering drugs."

"Even if earthlings can overcome their fear and

> **return to traditional foods," said the commission, "it will take centuries to repopulate the earth." The delegation expressed regret at the waste of a fine planet.**

I wish I'd written that.

Caveat emptor: Don't be misled by advertisements promising no cholesterol, low cholesterol or just a teensy weensy bit of cholesterol. Also pay no attention to food products promising to lower your cholesterol. Like cute, cuddly puppies, cholesterol is a marketing ploy.

Time to stick in a sidebar. You needed a martini, didn't you? A report by the National Academy of Sciences concludes that trans fatty acids are as bad as, maybe even worse than, saturated fats in raising heart disease risk. The NAS has concluded that trans fatty acids boost, yep, you guessed it, levels of "the most damaging form of cholesterol," the dreaded LDL. Worse (what could be worse?), trans fatty acids lower the levels of our good buddy HDL.

So there you have it from the experts. If you eat butter or any food that contains saturated fat, you'll raise your LDL cholesterol. However, if you try to eliminate foods that contain sat. fat by substituting products made from PUFAs, you'll raise your LDL levels. What's a person to do?

The Soy Ploy

Several years ago, a dieticians' darling made its debut. Finally after years of reluctantly placing meats, eggs, butter and cheese (God forbid!) in diets to provide the required amount of protein, diet planners had a safe (?) substitute. Out of what was once considered a waste product that would gag a maggot came a high-protein food product completely free of cholesterol (here we go again). The much-heralded debutante was soy, the miracle food that, aided by the FDA and mucho marketing, changed the eating habits of virtuous vegetarians, food faddists and diet disciples throughout the world.

The champagne has been flowing freely for soy advocates the past several years. Vegetarians danced in the streets after learning they could improve their protein intake without having to eat food products that came from something that had a mother (thank you, Mr. Rogers). Joy and jubilation among diet planners followed the USDA decision to allow unlimited use of soy in school lunches. Prior to that announcement, student meals were limited to 30% soy. Now, with soy added to hamburgers, tacos and lasagna, dieticians can get the total fat content below 30% and conform to government dictates thereby encouraging kids to bring their own lunch or go across the street to the fast food joint. For your information, a public relations firm hired by the soy industry successfully convinced the USDA to scrap the old soy limit.

Soy supporters are quick to let us know their sweetheart is more than a substitute for condiments from carnivores. According to Mark

Messina, a soy guru, "Each year, research on the health effects of soy and soybean components seems to increase exponentially. Furthermore, research is not just expanding in the primary areas under investigation, such as cancer, heart disease and osteoporosis; new findings suggest that soy has potential benefits that may be more extensive than previously thought." Indeed, in addition to preventing heart disease and staving off cancer, soy supposedly cools down hot flashes, builds strong bones and keeps us forever young. Future research will undoubtedly add boils, bunions and butt fungus to the list of ailments cured by Cinderella soy.

Little science and much marketing account for the success of soy. Had Mark Twain consumed but one serving of some soy product, the marketers would undoubtedly have attributed his talent, success and vitality to regular servings of soy. For more than a decade, marketing specialists had been busting their butts to gain consumer acceptance of tofu, soy milk, soy ice cream, soy cheese, soy sausage and soy derivatives, particularly soy isoflavones like genistein and diadzen, the estrogen-like compounds found in soybeans. The campaign was deemed a success when the Food and Drug Administration endorsed soy by deciding on October 25, 1999, to allow a health claim for products "low in saturated fat and cholesterol" that contain 6.25 grams of soy protein per serving. The declaration made it possible to claim any food is beneficial to cardiovascular health, as long as the product contains one heaping teaspoon of soy protein per 100-gram serving.

The folks at the FDA obviously need more lecithin, zinc, boron and a whole lot of other brain foods in their diets because the legality of adding soy protein to diets is questionable. Although soy protein has been approved for use as a binder in cardboard boxes, it has never been granted GRAS (generally regarded as safe) status for food. Imagine, the key ingredient of soy infant formula is not recognized as safe!

The lady is a tramp

Despite the hype and hullabaloo surrounding soy's ascent from the downtrodden stepsister to marrying the prince, several observations suggest the lady is a tramp. To begin with, soy's ability to prevent heart disease is dubious. After reviewing several studies with soy and discarding the ones that he didn't like, one soy scientist suggested that people who had cholesterol levels greater than 250 mg/dl (more metrics for you to ignore) could lower their cyclopentanoperhydrophenanthrene levels if they substituted soy protein for animal protein. *Caveat emptor* (that's Latin): if a person's cholesterol is less than 250 metric things, soy provides no benefits. Put simply, if your cholesterol is 249 metric things, then you might as well keep eating steak and burgers because soy won't help. The FDA's health claim doesn't mention this trivial detail.

Whether or not soy lowers cholesterol is unimportant. As sermonized earlier, there is no scientific evidence that lowering blood cholesterol prevents heart disease. Invoking the ambiguous cholesterol-lowering effect of soy is a part of the ploy to guide people to the grocery store aisle where soy products promise a life of health and vitality.

Speculation, and indeed it is speculation, that soy prevents cancer was fueled by a review of studies most of which involved animals. One study that showed soy caused pancreatic cancer in animals was overlooked but 65% of the other studies showed protective effects from soy. The studies with humans revealed mixed results, some indicated soy was protective but most showed no connection between eating soy and lowering cancer rates. While there is no sound evidence linking soy with lower incidence of cancer, the soy guru recommended one cup of soy products per day as part of a plan to prevent cancer.

More *caveat emptors*

Thousands of women are consuming soy hoping the overhyped product will protect them from breast cancer. Alas, two studies showed that soy protein and an ingredient of soy may promote breast cancer.

So as not to belabor the fact that soy has been over promoted and under studied, let me simply list some of the complaints lodged by concerned experts.

Soy is definitely not for the birds. After some exotic birds ate soy-based feed, the birds developed beautiful plumage several months earlier than expected. Unfortunately, the precocious maturation resulted in decreased fertility, beak and bone deformities, thyroid problems, immune malfunction and premature deaths. The problems were traced to a plant hormone found in the soy.

The FDA is well aware of problems associated with soy. Researchers with the FDA's National Center for Toxicological Research were very much embarrassed after discovering soy contains chemicals that interfere with the thyroid hormone.

Hot flashes are better than soy supplements. The smallest amount of soy protein claimed to lower cholesterol contains more than enough unsafe chemicals to block thyroid action.

Rather than keeping you young and vital, soy accelerates aging. Residents of Hawaii who ate more than two servings of tofu per week showed signs of accelerated brain aging. Those who had eaten tofu for a good part of their lives had a greater incidence of dementia and looked five years older than their ages. You're better off having three cocktails a day than eating soy (more about this later).

Soy is loaded with "antinutrients." Soy contains chemicals that block the action of enzymes needed to digest protein. Soy has the highest level of phytate (remember this scofflaw?) of any grain or legume studied. Monks used to drink soy milk (maybe they still do) to inhibit their sex desires.

Soy may rank with asbestos and tobacco. Like the manufacturers of asbestos and tobacco, the soy industry has denied any ill effects from consuming soy products. Perhaps the farmers who were persuaded to raise this miracle crop will be able to cash in on an increase in sales of boxes needed to ship and store the legal briefs that will be generated.

Diets

The term diet first showed up around 1200 AD. Back then and for many, many years, diet simply referred to what one was eating. Nowadays, when somebody talks about a diet, they are usually referring to a special concoction of foods and beverages that will help them lose weight. Diet has become synonymous with weight loss. This is a very common misconception. It isn't weight loss people desire, it's fat loss. However, because most diet plans do not result in fat loss, marketers refer to the plans as weight loss diets in order to keep their clients out of the courts.

Weight loss is okay to use because most of the diet programs succeed in this respect. The human body is about 75% water so anything that causes water loss will cause weight loss. But, *caveat emptor*, most diet programs don't turn the adipocytically challenged into the lithe and lean specimens of their dreams.

Diet plans have become prevalent because more people are becoming fat or worse, obese. According to the World Health Organization, obesity rates are doubling every 5-10 years. I'm not sure if that means people are getting twice as big every 5-10 years or twice as many people are getting obese. I suspect the latter. Every health professional in the world offers a reason for the increase in obesity but nobody knows for sure whose reason is right.

Many Ists blame the increase in obesity on the proliferation of ads touting unhealthy foods aimed at children. Back in 1970, the Federal Trade Commission tried to regulate advertising directed toward children but Congress put a stop to that. Since then, according to the experts, obesity rates have skyrocketed. There are other possibilities to consider. For example, because of budget restraints, many schools have cut physical education and nutrition programs. As a result, many kids aren't getting enough exercise and aren't learning about making food choices. When they make poor choices, experts blame the food. The successful banning of cigarette advertising has encouraged those who blame ads appealing to children. Look for future lawsuits to ban advertising of snacks and fast food.

One for Everybody

There are hundreds of diet plans for people to choose from, each promising significant success with a minimum of effort (otherwise they wouldn't be acceptable). Nothing causes more rancor in health professionals than the introduction of a new diet plan promising immediate restoration of health for the masses, unless of course the plan was devised by one of them. The animosity of professionals is often understandable since many of the "new and improved" diet plans have absolutely no research to back the claims. A vast majority of diets result from the fractured logic of the author and most are fact free.

Diet plans come with a variety of names and purposes. There are diets to prevent headaches, muscle aches, heartaches, bellyaches, toothaches and fungus—don't snicker at fungus, it's an underlying cause of many internal ailments. Some of the diets are named for the folks who devised them: the Atkins Diet, the Pritikin Diet, the Richard Simmons Diet and the Stillman Diet. Others are named for places: the Scarsdale Diet, the Scotsdale Diet, the I Love New York Diet, the I Love America Diet, the Beverly Hills Diet, the California Diet, the Mediterranean diet, the Himalayan Diet and the Puposky diet. Where the hell is Puposky? It's a community in northern Minnesota where my wife and I lived for 13 years and ate whatever we damn well pleased. One diet is named for the letter F and a recent diet wonders "What Would Jesus Eat?" The author of this plan claims that Christians and heathens alike could significantly improve their health by following Jesus' example.

Most of the folks who write diet books are a few bubbles from plumb. To devote even one sentence to each of the cockamamie diets in existence would require several volumes so this discussion will be limited to those that we can have the most fun with.

No or low carbs

The most talked about diets and the ones most popular with diet fans are the low-carbohydrate plans. The basic premise behind these programs is to eliminate carbohydrates from the diet and thereby keep insulin out of the blood. Insulin is an extremely important hormone but too much careening around blood vessels causes a lot of problems. Dr. Robert Atkins concocted the low-carb regimen that has been around the longest. This diet will cause bad breath.

Dr. Atkins forbids anything rich in carbohydrates including starchy vegetables and fruits. His strategy requires consumption of bacon and eggs, without hashbrowns and toast and cheeseburgers without the bun. Steaks are O.K. but forget the loaf of French bread. This diet is high in fat which forces the body to break down the fat in order to get the fuel it needs to heat the house and run the motors. Whenever fat is chewed up inside the body (metabolized is the fancy schmancy word), chemicals called ketones are made. Ketones, in a word, stink. Acetone is a ketone. Because acetone and other ketones are gases, they can be eliminated from the blood through the lungs. Folks who try this diet plan have breath that can level a landfill. Also, people trying this diet should never smoke or even lean over an open flame—acetone is highly flammable.

For people who believe low-carbohydrate diets are the answer to everlasting lithe but want to keep friends and work around flames, there are the low-carbohydrate, high-protein diets like the one fostered by Dr. and Dr. Eades (Mary and Michael). An Internet interview introduced the Eades as Dr. Michael Eades, MD and Dr. Mary Eades,

MD. Is that redundant or are they married dieticians? Then again, they're probably just a paradox.

The Eades' plan lets you eat fruits and vegetables so you won't stop a train with your breath but—like Atkins—steers you away from pasta, bread, cereals and rice. Although Atkins and the Eades are medical doctors, neither of these diets or any of the similar spin-offs are endorsed by a large majority of health professionals. Undaunted by scorn and criticism their creators just shrug their shoulders and claim it's politics—the sugar and wheat councils, after all, have strong lobbyists.

??? diets

There are a couple of diets that were allegedly devised by members of prestigious organizations, namely the American Medical Association (AMA) and Mayo Clinic. The AMA denies having anything to do with the so called AMA diet and takes no credit for its success or failure. The Mayo Clinic Diet is also a myth probably designed by somebody who likes mayonnaise. Why do so many people call it manaze?

Many foods contain ingredients that either melt fat or start the fire, at least according to the authors of the Grapefruit Diet, the Cottage Cheese Diet, the Banana Diet, the Oil Diet, the Cabbage Soup Diet and the Vinegar Diet. According to the Oil Diet lady, obesity is linked to environmental pollution so to lose weight (there's that term again) you have to detoxify your body. You do this by taking a swig of canola or olive oil, straight up, every day. I'm serious.

The Grapefruit Diet (a.k.a. the New Mayo Clinic Diet) has you eating anything you want at any meal until you are full or cannot eat anymore. (Is there a difference?) You must have grapefruit though because that is the catalyst that starts the fat burning. Can't you just hear the adipose cells sizzling and crackling as they burn up? No wonder the Ists get rancors. The instructions for the diet say it's important to eliminate sugars and starches, which are lipids and form fat. Excuse me, sugars and starches are carbohydrates. These people either color way outside of the lines or they're putting us on.

Cabbage soup everyday for seven days and you're guaranteed a loss of 10 to 15 pounds. Note, there's nothing here about how much fat you will lose. Nor is there anything said about the flatulence factor. Seven days on nothing but cabbage soup would undoubtedly lead to serious bloating accompanied by gas leakage.

And then there are apple cider vinegar pills. A pill a day melts the mush away. Isn't it time to add some more chlorine to the gene pool?

More Diets

Not all diets were devised for fat loss alone. Some are supposed to forever keep you free of disease. Barry Sears, Ph.D. who invites us to live in another dimension by entering "The Zone," devised a very popular diet that fits this category. In Sears' world, one is required to eat foods that supply energy from 40% carbohydrate, 30 % fat and 30% protein. Like others, Sears—no relation to Roebuck—is concerned about insulin but his formulation for eternal beauty and life is really a mid-carbohydrate diet rather than low-carb.

One of Dr. Sears' most insightful deductions is the fact that eating grains makes cows fat so the same would be true with humans. Isn't that enough to make you moderate your carbohydrate intake? As if it wasn't enough to insult cows by putting them in a category with humans, Sears inflamed coaches and athletes at Stanford University by taking credit for the success of the women's swim team. According to Sears, team members were put on his program and soon after defeated the University of Texas, thus ending a long series of losses to the Lady Longhorns. Sears didn't mention the fact that the Texas swim coach, along with several outstanding athletes, had transferred to Stanford. Do you want to follow a program devised by a man who insulted cows and then talented, dedicated coaches and athletes?

As of this writing Sears has not published any research data in a scientific journal nor has any reputable health organization even acknowledged Sears' program. His book, however, is selling which goes to show the measures people go to hoping to find health's holy grail.

What you don't know about ABO

Do you know your blood type? Most people don't and if you're one of those you'd better run down to the local clinic to have your blood typed. While you're there, give a pint. That was a public service announcement. Will that qualify me for some kind of benefits?

A diet that surfaced in 1996 gives a whole new meaning to blood typing. Previously it was necessary to know a person's blood type (A,B, AB,O) to prevent mishaps during emergency blood transfusions. Giving B blood to an A type would be disastrous!

Now, according to the author of the blood-type diet, it's disastrous for a person to eat without knowing their blood type. For example, milk is absolutely verboten for the Type A individual. Drink milk, A guy, and your blood will agglutinate (glob together) and you'll die of a brain hemorrhage with a silly milk mustache on your face.

Folks with Type O blood are flirting with danger if they eat beans, legumes or anything made from wheat. According to the author, if you eat a bowl of bean chili, proteins from the beans overpower your muscles, altering their function and diminishing your physical capabilities. Now I understand why there is so much flatulence accompanying a good chili dinner—the ol' sphincter muscles have been done in by the beans.

Along with chili beans, Type O folks are warned to never, ever, eat any kind of whole-wheat products. Have you ever been at a restaurant when the man in the booth across from you takes a bite of whole-wheat bread and suddenly spews his half-digested salad and meatloaf all over his mate seated across from him? Neither have I, but it might happen if you don't follow the blood type guidelines.

As if upchucking a meal containing wheat products isn't enough, the author tells us Type O folks can't produce enough iodine. Now that is serious business. Imagine, just because a person has inherited the genes for making Type O blood, they can't produce enough iodine to make their thyroid gland work efficiently. Come to think of it, nobody produces iodine. Matter of fact, nobody produces potassium or calcium or magnesium or zinc or germanium. Iodine and all the others are nutrients that are gotten only by eating food!

The blood-type expert obviously thinks the chemicals on red blood cells (these are the gas bags that carry oxygen to the cells and carbon dioxide away from cells) are extremely influential because they supposedly help determine personality traits. According to the author, people with Type A blood are docile, submissive, tofu eating vegetarians who can't deal with pressure and could never be President of the United States or the CEO of a company producing and selling tofu. The Type B eats about anything, loves dairy products and likes to be seen sporting a silly milk mustache. Type O individuals are, according to the expert, flesh eating, dominant, caveman types who are the epitome of strength, endurance, self reliance, daring, intuition and just about everything Hitler was looking for in a master race. Hitler, by the way, would have ended up in one of his ovens if blood testing had come into vogue during his reign of terror; he was, according to the author, a mutated Type A personality.

Widespread acceptance of the ABO diet could lead to a glut of specialty stores cropping up around the nation. Al's Type A Cuisine, We Cater to Wimps. Bud's Type B Market, The Store for the Omnivore. Jessie's Type O Butcher Shop, Where Everything is Flesh. If the FDA decided to take the blood type diet seriously—which is highly unlikely, but then you never know about those folks—food labels would have to include a statement indicating who can buy the product. Also, to prevent accidental vomiting or death, the purchaser would have to show appropriate ID at the counter.

The foreign diet

The Mediterranean Diet is the last one I'm going to mention, although there are many more out there. While surfing the Internet, I learned that the Mediterranean Diet has its own pyramid. Apparently a gang of Mediterraneans enslaved a bunch of people who didn't care for the food (probably goofy Germans) and made them construct a pyramid. It's located in Greece, not to be confused with grease, which is a lipid (a.k.a. fat). Unlike the Pyramids of Beltsville, the Mediterranean Pyramid has a foundation upon which the pyramid sits. The foundation is daily physical exercise. You are required to swim the Mediterranean, shore to shore, every day, after which you can drink six glasses of water and two glasses of wine.

The lower chamber of the pyramid is filled with bread, pasta, rice, couscous, polenta, other grains and potatoes. On the door to this chamber is a sign informing us that this and the next three passages are called the daily chambers. The next level is divided into three separate rooms containing fruits, beans, legumes and nuts and vegetables. In the hall above, olives are strewn about the floor and bottles filled with olive oil line the shelves. Cheese and yogurt occupy all the space in the chamber over the oil.

Ascending up to the next level, one finds a sign reading "Entering the Weekly Chambers." The first is filled with fish which are beginning to smell a little, the next has poultry running around so you have to be careful where you step. Above the poultry is a room filled with nests holding fresh eggs. There is a candy store called "Sweets" above the egg room. A flight of stairs leads to the top of the pyramid but a gate keeps us from going up. The proprietor of the candy store informs us the top chamber is filled with meat but can be visited only once a month.

Although the Mediterranean Diet contains as much as 40% of total Calories from fat, it is apparently acceptable to most nutrition scientists because the fat is olive oil which doesn't raise cholesterol (spare me). Some experts claim the Mediterranean Diet is healthier than the American diet. (Which one?) The American Heart Association acknowledges that the incidence of heart disease is lower in Mediterranean countries but "more research is needed."

Confusing the Consumer

Fat

There are many things nutrition experts disagree on, the most recent being how much fat should be in a diet. After years of proselytizing the benefits of a low-fat diet, the American Heart Association reversed its position when they told consumers the fat content of their diets should be greater than 15% of total Calories. Is it any wonder the average consumer reads books like this one for advice about nutrition?

Since the American Heart Association is a prestigious group made up of people who take zinc, boron and lecithin supplements, lipophobics were insulted and outraged. "Traitors!" they exclaimed and took to the streets chanting slogans like, "AHA means America's Hardened Arteries," and "The fatter you're fed, the sooner you're dead." They also invoked the cute, cuddly puppy by reminding us "everybody knows low-fat diets lead to reduced cholesterol."

The American Heart Association's answer to the critics was, "Some very low-fat diets showed impressive heart disease risk reducing results, but more research is needed."

Regardless of what the AHA or any other group of decision makers decide, a psychology professor at Yale University, recognized as a leading expert on obesity (an obesitist?), has proposed the ideal solution to world's pudgy problem: a fat tax. The prof suggests we treat high-fat foods as luxury items like tobacco and alcohol. The profits from the tax would, of course, go to nutrition education and physical fitness programs.

In addition to a luxury tax on fat foods, other regulations should be imposed. Tobacco and alcohol can't be sold to individuals under a specified age so we should require similar regulations for the sale of high-fat food. To begin with, all high-fat foods will be kept on locked shelves surrounded by wire fencing. To purchase a high-fat food, an individual will have to submit to a body mass test. Weighing would never suffice because muscle is heavier than fat so a tall, muscular individual might not pass the test even though they have only 5% body fat.

For the program to work and work effectively, everybody is going to have to have body fat measured on the spot. We don't want any fake or outdated identification being presented. The difficulty is going to be deciding on an acceptable body fat. This will undoubtedly bring heated debate in Congress. "He's not too fat to fight for his country, why can't he buy a T-bone steak?" There will also be a need for fat policemen who will insist on being referred to as lipid lawmen. Stiff fines will be imposed on obese people caught purchasing fat foods and on those caught selling fat food to the adipocytically challenged.

Two for one

Who would ever believe that an airline could do something to help fight the problem of obesity? I know what you're thinking: airline food—an oxymoron—encourages abstention. But that's not what I'm referring to. Southwest Airlines, prompted by complaints from customers, has decided to enforce a policy requiring "customers of size" (a.k.a. fat asses) to buy two seats. With this policy in effect, passengers who are too large to squeeze between the armrests of one seat will have to buy another ticket for their butts.

Several airlines have had the policy in effect for years but haven't enforced it. This was due in part to the fact that, in the past, many flights were not filled. With the cutback in flights this is no longer the case and irate customers—tired of sharing their seats with overhanging flab from larger neighbors—have begun complaining.

The "customers of size" policy brought immediate protest from the adipocitically challenged along with the organization that defends them. Did you know the obese have a protecting organization? Yep. The Obesity Law and Advocacy Center located in San Diego. "To take this position regardless of whether or not a flight is filled is reprehensible," whined one of the founders of OLAC. "There's no reason to charge anyone if there's room available."

"We're tired of being pinned down by their overflow," countered a satisfied Southwest customer.

When other airlines begin enforcing the oversize policy, expect some major flight delays. In order to determine whether or not a large person is truly a two-seater, the airlines are going to have to install a regulation airplane seat at each check-in counter. They'll be called "assess seats." If a clerk suspects a customer needs two seats, the suspect will be required to sit in the chunky checker. Flight delays will undoubtedly occur because of the need to call in emergency crews to extricate the really rotund.

Fat breaks

Not to be out done by airlines taking measures that would help alleviate the obesity problem in the country, the government has also stepped in to slow sloth. The Internal Revenue Service (a.k.a. IRS) is now offering a tax break to Americans who are willing to control their weight. In April of 2002 the IRS, recognizing that obesity is a disease (and you thought they were all a bunch of dimwitted accountants), said that it would begin allowing taxpayers to claim weight loss expenses as a medical deduction. Previously taxpayers could deduct costs of weight loss programs as a medical expense **only** if they were recommended by a doctor to treat a specific disease. Obesity now qualifies as a disease.

We Americans are very creative when it comes to tax deductions and it doesn't take too much zinc or lecithin to realize that fruits, vegetables, low-fat milk and for that matter lean meats all contribute to loss of body fat. Thus, the disgustingly lithe (and probably vain) person who thinks they are "so fat" could conceivably deduct their entire yearly food bill along with their bicycles, special clothing and trips to the gym under the guise of weight loss. Americans spend more than $30 billion a year on weight loss products or programs. That coupled with some creativity during tax preparation could mean a significant decrease in tax revenues, which could result in decreased government spending (heaven forbid).

The gesture on the part of the IRS is indeed benevolent but to prevent fat fraud will necessitate the use of another tax form, that being Form 6-1-20 (F is the sixth letter in the alphabet, A the first, etc.). The IRS is going to have to know just how much fat one is packing around and how much was actually lost before they start letting individuals go off willy nilly deducting the costs of weight loss. To accomplish this, they will probably include the simple (this is the IRS we're talking about) and very popular formula for calculating one's BMI. "What do my bowel movements have to do with fat?" you ask. Nothing, this is the Body Mass Index, which is supposed to tell you whether or not you are adipocytically challenged.

Fat formula

This is how it works: holding a pencil in the hand you commonly write with (left-handed people are supposedly smarter that righties but right-handed people live a few years longer), back up to a wall, place the pencil on the top of your head with the point toward the wall and make a mark on the wall. Next, measure the distance in inches from the floor to the mark (you'd probably better write this number down somewhere so you don't forget and mislead the IRS). Now, go weigh yourself and truthfully write down the number of pounds the scale registers. By now you've probably lost a couple of pounds from exertion so you'd better go have a bacon cheeseburger with fries and reweigh immediately after. Remember, you want the IRS to think you have a disease.

After obtaining your height in inches and your weight in pounds, it's time to do some arithmetic. Don't worry, your calculator can handle these operations. First determine the square of your height. If you've forgotten how to get the square or failed elementary math, you simply multiply your height (in inches) times your height (in inches). Now, divide your weight in pounds by the square of your height and *voila,* you have a number that you're supposed to multiply times 703 (I have no idea where 703 comes from. It's not a Fibonacci number and 700 would make us less fat). After the marking, weighing and arithmeticing, you are ready to see if you are fat or not. If the number you arithmeticed is less than 25 you are lissome, healthy and probably lying. If the number you got is 25 to 29, you are skillful with a pencil, ruler and scale and truthful because that's what over a third of our nation is—overweight. If your number is 30 or above you buy your clothes at the local tent and awning or soon will. As you can see from the BMI formula, only 30's and above qualify for Form 6-1-20. Unfortunately, over a fourth of our country falls in this category of being obese (soon to be known as adipocytically challenged). Look for a marked decrease in tax revenue as a result of a marked increase in fat tissue. Also, the tax auditor of the future will be armed with a tape measure and scale.

Another Fat Unveiled

According to the Center for Science in the Public Interest (CSPI), a fast food watchdog group that really aggravates most consumers (that's us, the folks who buy food or PEOPLE), there are actually two kinds of saturated fats. After condemning several fast foods and theater popcorn, the CRAPS, oops, the CSPI tested several kinds of pizza before they stuffed their faces with the scrumptious slices. The tests revealed that two or three slices of plain cheese pizza contain 25 metric things of fat, including ten metric things of **artery-clogging** saturated fat. So there you have it. The people who watch what we eat and probably eat the same things have discovered a second kind of saturated fat. The president of Pizza Hut reacted to this new discovery with: "Americans love cheese. We respond to the voice of our customer. And frankly, I think people are a little tired of being told what not to eat."

So, thank you very much, you CSPIs, for enlightening us about that new kind of fat. And, since you're the same bunch who told us a few years back that buttered popcorn should be avoided, listen up 'cause we have news for you. Researchers have discovered that popcorn might help prevent insulin resistance, a disorder that leads to type 2 diabetes. Type 2 is the kind of diabetes that develops because of poor diet and lack of exercise. Professionals once referred to it as "adult onset diabetes" but lately it has been showing up in teenagers so they had to take out the adult part. Type 2 diabetes is increasing at an alarming rate and the practitioners aren't sure why. It probably has to due with the fact people aren't getting enough exercise and the CSPIs keep condemning foods long before researchers have a chance to test and condone them.

Also, some group once condemned dairy foods. I'm not sure who—probably the CSPIs. Like popcorn, researchers now think dairy foods help prevent the development of insulin resistance.

And let's not forget peanut butter. Once condemned as a heart beater, research has shown that this scrumptious sandwich filler helps shrink adipocytes.

Salt

Salt was a newsworthy item thousand of years before health experts started bickering about it. The headlines of an ancient scroll read, "Armed Bandits Raid Salt Caravan." The story tells how masked men, carrying state-of-the-art swords and spears, stopped a caravan and carried off all the salt. Another scroll describes how the greedy Huntius brothers tried to corner the salt market by buying all available stores and hoarding it on their property beside the Dead Sea. Unfortunately for the Huntius boys, a rainstorm dissolved their cache leaving them broke and destitute and the Dead Sea saturated with salt. Still another scroll headline tells of Roman soldiers striking for higher salt.

Before technology made it otherwise, salt was in short supply and therefore a precious commodity. Caravans loaded with salt traveled hundreds of miles to trade for gold and fine linens. Soldiers were often paid with salt, giving rise to the term "salary." In the Middle Ages, spilling salt was thought to be a sign of impending doom. That was before ladders, mirrors and black cats were invented. Our ancestors recognized simple salt as a valuable chemical for cleaning, dyeing, softening leather, bleaching and preserving meat. They also realized it was an important part of their diets and worth trading and sometimes slitting a throat for.

Although salt is now easily obtainable and affordable, this simple compound, sodium chloride, continues to remain a newsworthy item because scientists can't agree on its impact on health. After years of being told salt causes high blood pressure and heart disease, and paying little attention to the decree, the public was overjoyed to learn a study had proved that a low-salt diet caused heart disease. Housewives and gourmet cooks breathed a sigh of relief as they pushed their collection of exotic spices to the back of the pantry. Congress debated whether or not to declare a "Salt is Safe" holiday, increasing the number of yearly days off for federal workers to 200.

The joy that swept through the land was soon dampened by the proclamation that "more research is needed." Revelers put away their noisemakers and pointed hats and went back to bland tasting food until another momentous announcement was made—studies show there is little or no correlation between salt intake and blood pressure. Again, joy and happiness reigned supreme as chefs flavored their carefully crafted creations in the kitchen with more than a pinch of salt while patrons—without even tasting first—shook more flavor onto their servings. Meanwhile scientists lamented to unhearing hordes, "more research is needed."

This whole controversial mess with salt started about 6,000 to 8,000 years ago when our distant relatives went from picking nuts and berries and slaying wooly mammoths to cultivating crops and raising pigs and cows. To survive, they needed to preserve and to stockpile foods for the long winter months when they played

Monopoly and hanky panky.

Vegetables and meats were dried until somebody discovered adding salt could preserve food. Our forefathers and foremothers quickly realized adding salt to food did more than kill the little bugs slithering around in their rations. Salt adds flavor and heightens existing flavors, even in sweets; a whole new dimension had been added to the pleasures of eating. "Please pass the salt."

Neither the USDA nor the FDA wants to put a number on how much salt we should eat. These agencies hope that people will choose diets that contain moderate amounts of salt. This is nice but folks need some kind of number to know if their diets are modest or immodest.

The National Research Council of the National Academy of Sciences doesn't believe the reports that say there is no connection between salt intake and health. This scholarly bunch had some meetings, took some votes and determined that the recommended safe minimum daily amount is about 500 metric things of sodium with an upper limit of 2,400. Completely disregarding the reports about salt and health, the council has said that lowering sodium intake to 1,800 metric things would probably be healthier. They're probably right but "more research is needed."

Fish Stories

First the experts told to us to eat copious (that's a big word) quantities of fish to stay healthy and then they rescinded and told us not to eat too much or we would turn into giant guppies. Fish contains EFAs and PUFAs that our bodies need to make important chemicals, and people who eat fish smell bad. No, actually they have less heart disease. According to a brief overview published in an American Dietetic Association's Nutrition in Complementary Care newsletter, omega-3 fatty acids (EFAs) "are believed to contribute to an overall vascular environment less prone to occlusion by atherosclerotic plaques." This, of course, made everybody want to eat more fish.

While folks were rushing to health food stores looking for fish oils or crowding into fish markets to buy the real thing, somebody did an experiment and discovered that some EFAs and PUFAs get in the way of others and muck up production schedules in the body. This prompted a warning against eating too much fish. That's the science story. The real truth is wives started complaining that their husbands were spending far too much time fishing after the first "eat more fish" proclamation. Give a man a fish and he will eat for a day. Teach a man how to fish and he'll sit in a boat and drink beer all day.

Never to be outdone at making rules and regulations, the Environmental Protection Agency (EPA), an organization that worries a lot about our health, agreed it's not a good idea to eat more than two fish a week. They are concerned people who eat a lot of fish will get too much mercury in their systems. At a symposium in California some EPA who-hahs announced that 89% of people who eat fish every day have high levels of mercury in their bodies. The people who attended the conference were so upset by the proclamation that most of them ordered fish for dinner that night.

If you don't live near a stream, river, lake or the ocean you can buy two fish a week at the supermarket to get your needs. If you hate fish, use canola oil, flaxseed, walnuts, or wheat germ. Supplements are another option but be sure they contain at least two fish a week. These numbers are subject to change and undoubtedly will.

Alcohol

For years alcohol was forbidden in the diet so the experts didn't have to argue about it. Then, along came a study saying a couple of drinks of wine every day might be healthy but it had to be red wine. After scientists discovered some antioxidants in red wine it was not only posh to have a glass or two with dinner, it was actually healthy. Of course, there are a few of those who think if some's good, more's better and they nearly ruined it for the rest of us by drinking three or four glasses. Aristocrats were bummed because it's totally gauche to drink red wine with fish and other healthy white meats but then somebody found antioxidants in white wine and the gentry was appeased.

Health addicts were guzzling their fine wines and turning up their noses at folks who like a cocktail or two before dinner until a study showed that one or two alcoholic drinks a day of any kind might be healthy. While I was working on this masterpiece, scientists reported that three drinks a day of wine, beer, or distilled spirits not only protects us from heart disease and stroke but also prevents Alzheimer's disease and other types of dementia. Now I remember why my wife and I started having a couple of gin and tonics for an evening cocktail.

Nuts to You

Just a few years ago, if you had skipped up to an Ist and said, "Please, please, oh learned sage, tell me which snack is the heart healthiest: a package of nuts, a chocolate bar, a package of pretzels, or a bag of chips?" the expert would first regard you the way a Parisian waiter regards an American tourist who pronounces croissant as if the breakfast roll were the grumpy sister of a parent, and then blurt, "Pretzels, of course, they're lowest in fat." Not so today. The pretzels are still the lowest in fat but the Ist would tell you nuts are the healthiest because they contain healthy fat not that nasty saturated fat that raises the demon cholesterol.

Although the experts once censured nuts, now they are lauded for being not only a good source of magnesium, vitamin E and fiber (better than grasshoppers) but unsaturated fats as well. According to the Ists, five big studies have found that folks who eat nuts have less chance of getting heart disease. Furthermore, the experts are happy to announce that "several clinical studies have found heart-healthy diets containing various nuts or peanuts to be beneficial in lowering total and LDL cholesterol in study participants." Now, aren't you sorry you gave up eating nuts back when the experts told us they weren't healthy because they contained too much fat?

Just how healthy are nuts? When 86,000 nurses were followed for 14 years and 22,000 physicians were studied for 11 years, the people who ate the most nuts were less likely to die from heart disease according to the Ists who studied the studies. First of all, what were those nurses and doctors doing eating nuts when they were supposed to be harmful? Don't professionals listen to what other professionals tell them? Second, the folks who ate the nuts had lower cholesterol levels, which prompted the experts to **claim** they were less likely to get heart disease.

So, if you still believe the cuddly puppy propaganda about cholesterol, eat more than a half cup of nuts every week. Even if you don't believe in good cholesterol and bad cholesterol, eat nuts regularly. They're good for you and the Ists won't care because the Calories come from the good unsaturated fat. But don't over do it unless you're looking for another tax deduction.

More Confusion

A few months ago, a science reporter was frantically perusing the wire services in search of a riveting story about food and nutrition. Desperately he tried to find a story about a nutrient that caused cancer or a nutrient that prevented cancer or how soy prevents halitosis, herpes and heartburn or a report that soy causes dandruff or body hair and sometimes both dandruff and body hair or a study proving fish oil makes boogers and ear wax softer or results showing that anybody who has the teeny weenyist amount of cholesterol in their blood is bound to die, sometime. Tirelessly he combed the news reports frenetically seeking anything that he could sensationalize and make a story to satisfy his editor. But alas, there was nothing startling or even new coming out of the citadels of science so he was obliged to dig through old files to find something newsworthy.

On that slow news day, our reporter chose as his topic for confusion the interactions among vitamins and minerals. With riveting prose he reported that calcium might decrease the absorption of iron, zinc, and magnesium. That insightful information was followed by the statement that iron might decrease the absorption of zinc, calcium, copper and manganese which was followed by the report that zinc might inhibit copper absorption. Can't you picture these essential minerals in mortal hand to hand combat at the gates of the intestine battling to gain entry into the blood? Makes you wonder how we ever survived as a species. Not to worry, faithful readers (I say faithful because you've endured this far), the interactions outlined by our dutiful reporter are not life threatening. They are, in fact, nugatory (if you're not sure, look it up and I think you'll agree this was a good word choice for this section).

Back in the days when Ists liked to study interactions among vitamins and minerals (that's no longer fashionable) they would pick a vitamin or mineral they thought might do some interacting and feed it to caged rodents in quantities that would keep a water buffalo healthy. Then they tested the rodents' pee and poop to see if some vitamins and minerals were being bullied around. As you might expect, some were. However, the results were never very meaningful because the amount of interacter being fed was several times the daily requirement of the rodents and none of the vitamins and minerals in the diet were added in the form actually found in food. For example, when somebody reported that calcium interfered with zinc, they weren't talking about calcium being bottle fed to rodents in the form of milk. And the zinc wasn't hooked on to picolinate or some other amino acid or protein. The experiments simply weren't what happens on a day to day basis in real life in real humans.

Even though the interacting studies were useless, nutrition scientists kept grinding them out (you've heard of publish or perish) so now we have a whole bunch of irrelevant interactions that science reporters can dredge up on the days somebody hasn't discovered a food product that will prevent toe jam. Here are a few more gems that our distressed scribe culled from the archives of irrelevant data. Dairy foods, due to their high content of phosphorus, might reduce calcium absorption. Just remember, dairy foods have been proven to be excellent sources of calcium in humans and that's what we are, I think. You know nutritious discoveries were lacking when you read the part where the correspondent tells us vitamin D is needed for the most efficient absorption of calcium. That's pretty common knowledge these days. You also know the writer isn't an Ist when he tells us that folks who take calcium supplements should also take vitamin D supplements. Ists don't recommend supplements. According to the article, regular use of folic acid might decrease zinc levels in the body so zinc supplements may be helpful. Nutrition experts constantly remind us of the importance of folic acid and some have even suggested supplements (more sacrilege) but I've never witnessed one inviting zinc supplements as well. Also, this one is confusing because folic acid is supposed to improve brain function, zinc is also very important to the 'ol cerebral cells.

Vitamin C may decrease the absorption of copper but increase the absorption of iron. That last part is meaningful so we won't make fun of it. The first part was the impetus for my first medical mystery, "Beyond Containment," but when it turned out to be laughable (the first part, not the book), I had to make some major changes in the plot. Buy the novel, read it and then you'll understand.

In his report, our journalist was particularly hard on coffee, informing us that coffee increases calcium loss, which may lead to bone loss and osteoporosis. According to a report from the National Institutes for Health, fat, phosphorous, magnesium and caffeine do not affect calcium absorption or excretion significantly. While the article claims coffee also inhibits iron absorption along with zinc absorption, there are no studies proving coffee consumption leads to iron deficiency or a weakened immune system or memory loss.

Antiaging

In the past, many Ists talked and wrote about the antiaging properties of certain foods (fruits and vegetables, obviously). Nowadays they will do so under the threat of being criticized as a heretic. Fifty-one scientists got so upset with the burgeoning anti-aging "scam" that they wrote and endorsed a position paper, which can be found on the *Scientific American* website (at least when this book went to press it was there). In their own words, "The researchers who wrote and endorsed the position paper don't necessarily agree on every word written there, but…" (surprise, surprise). According to the experts who drafted the document, "There has been a resurgence and proliferation of health care providers and entrepreneurs who are promoting antiaging products and lifestyle changes that they claim will slow, stop or reverse the processes of aging. Even though in most cases there is little or no scientific basis for these claims, the public is spending vast sums of money on these products and lifestyle changes, some of which may be harmful. Scientists are unwittingly contributing to the proliferation of these pseudoscientific antiaging products by failing to participate in the public dialogue about the genuine science of aging research." Reminded me of the cholesterol scam.

A couple of months after publication of the temper tantrum by the "fed-up fifty-one," *Scientific American* published an interesting article describing how a technique called caloric restriction has worked remarkably well in prolonging the life of experimental animals. What was it Mark Twain said about scientists and their theories?

Crud From Cows

When I was young and my mother sent me to the store to buy margarine, I came home with a bag of white glob that had a little yellow orb in the middle. I pressed on the yellow gob until it oozed out into the white stuff and then I squeezed and pinched and kneaded until all the white stuff had turned yellow. The white stuff was a PUFA called margarine, which was chock full of trans fatty acids. The yellow dye, of course, was needed to make the margarine look like butter. Later, the manufactures started putting the dye in the PUFAs and kids didn't have the fun of poking the bag of glob anymore. Later still, some scientists began to wonder if those trans fatty acids, which the body doesn't make or recognize, might be doing some harm. Health professionals, who had for years been preaching the dangers of the saturated fats in butter said, "Oops!" and suddenly began telling us to use half real butter and half margarine. During the past few years we've learned those harmful saturated fats are needed to sustain a healthy life.

Milk became the center of controversy several years ago when a well-known scientist suggested that the secretions from a cow's udder contain a protein that annoys our immune systems and causes them to destroy the pancreas leading to diabetes. That was determined to be a bunch of poppycock but there were still those who whined about the saturated fats in the milk and told us to get our daily calcium needs by eating truckloads of vegetables. A few months ago newspapers and magazines carried headlines telling us we could lose weight by eating a common everyday food, which turns out to be none other than milk. According to recent research results, milk contains a chemical that causes adipocytes (see glossary) to release their stored goods. Also, calcium, found in milk, is needed so that cells can toss out fat (a.k.a. lipid).

On the subject of calcium, we find there's some confusion and controversy. Since calcium is the most abundant mineral in our bodies, men and women are encouraged to consume 1000 to 1300 metric things per day. However, according to a recent Harvard survey, men who get more than 600 metric things a day have a higher risk of prostate cancer. I wish I could remember the name of the person who stated "Life is just one damn carcinogen after another," so I could give him proper credit.

Supplements

Dateline Grand Forks, ND (across the river from East Grand Forks, MN).

An expert from the USDA Grand Forks Human Nutrition Research Center was told a common reason why many people consider supplements is because they have been led to believe that our farming land, hence food supply, is nutrient depleted. The expert disagreed stating that the current food sources "...are still full of all the "good" nutrients."

Dateline Beltsville, MD

A senior research scientist with the USDA Agricultural Research Service stated that few foods provide more than 10 to 15 percent of the minimum suggested chromium intake.

The USDA "expert" in North Dakota obviously doesn't consider chromium one of the "good" nutrients (he probably believes in good and bad cholesterol too). According to the USDA (that's the agency that built the lab west of East Grand Forks and, using our tax money, pays the salary of the resident "experts"), four ounces of spinach contains about three metric things of iron. If that valuable piece of information doesn't excite you, wait until you read that the same amount of spinach contained more than 150 metric things back in 1948. That's only a fifty-fold loss in fifty years. At that rate, another few years and Popeye will have to take iron supplements. But the current food sources "...are still full of all the "good" nutrients." Our North Dakota expert is full of something and it isn't "good" nutrients.

FYI: In the mid 90s one of the "experts" at the North Dakota lab wrote a treatise in which he stated that chromium is not essential for humans. A few months later, after considering several clinical studies, higher officials within the USDA determined that chromium is an essential nutrient for humans.

Little wonder the average consumer is confused about supplements when they're hearing opposing views from people in the same agency. But then, experts have been confusing consumers about food supplements since the first vitamin/mineral pills became available.

When the supplement industry was a fledgling, every health professional spurned supplements, especially physicians who knew virtually nothing about nutrition or food supplements. In those days, physicians were trained to cure disease, usually with drugs, and there was very little evidence to convince them supplements had any redeeming qualities. Prevention was not in their vocabularies.

As Peter, Paul and Mary told us, "The times they are a changin'." Because of careful research and documentation, a steadily increasing number of health professionals are beginning to recognize the value of food supplements. Unfortunately, a large cadre of authorities continually claims "you can get what you need from a balanced diet."

The "eat a balanced diet" preachers apparently took courses in money management and divinity while studying to become Ists. From their pious pulpits they berate supplements as a waste of money. In their sanctimonious writings and lectures, they tell us to get our nutrients from food and not pills.

The religion and banking classes must have conflicted with courses in reality. A well-balanced diet chock full of nutrient-rich fruits and vegetables is certainly a well-balanced idea but in our society it just ain't going to happen. Convenience and satiety sabotage resolute resolutions and sincere strategies. "I'd like to eat healthier food but fast food is easy and tastes good."

Abbreviated breakfasts, lunch, dinner and fast food emporiums have replaced Mom's and Grandma's home cooked delicacies. "Mom, don't put anything in the microwave for me tonight, I'll have a burger at E. Coli's after practice."

Clever marketing entices us to tantalize our taste buds with not-so-nutritious cuisine. And then there are those of us who don't like vegetables. My friend Jack Challem says, "It's harder to give up bad eating habits than tobacco."

As if the lure of non-nutritious foods isn't bad enough, we have the problem of latitude, longitude and a thing called seasons. Fresh nutrient-rich fruits and vegetables aren't available year round in every locale. Rather than religion and banking, the budding experts should have taken a course in geography.

They're cheap and easy

Oh yes, and then there is that age-old problem of age. In a column by a Ph.D., R.D. Ist, the writer stated, "Unfortunately, it's sometimes difficult for older adults to consume the variety of foods and nutrients that are needed to stay healthy." She went on to tell the old duffers that they couldn't taste or smell things like they could back when they were young whipper snappers so they needed to add some spice to their life by adding spice to their food. And be sure you chew it well, which may be difficult, because seniors often have oral health problems, but never mind, your dentist can take care of that.

The expert stated that she couldn't understand why so many old folks don't have an appetite. Back in the 1970s a talented researcher showed that loss of zinc in the diet led to a loss of appetite. Apparently the lady cut class the day the prof talked about that. The expert blamed digestive problems, medications, anxiety, loneliness and depression and suggested eating four to six smaller meals, preferably when they weren't napping. Also she suggested avoiding foods that will make you fart.

Our well educated Ist got in the part about fruits and vegetables by informing the oldsters their digestive systems have gotten feeble so they might have trouble pooping. However, eight glasses of water a day (that's a lot of oxy gin and hydro gin), along with those high-fiber fruits and veggies will have you producing on the pot once again.

Let's be sure we're clear on this. If older people get their teeth fixed, eat spicy but not too spicy food, watch humorous videos with friends or read humorous books (like this one), drink eight glasses of water a day and eat fruits and vegetables six times a day, they'll get the nutrients they need. Not once did the expert suggest that older adults need food supplements to fortify their nutrient intake so they might have an appetite and enjoy eating.

Without doubt, every nutritional scientist in the world agrees that people should be encouraged to eat fruits and vegetables. A good many of those also realize it won't happen soon. According to a survey conducted at UC Berkeley a few years ago, only 9% of the population ate three to five daily servings of fruits and vegetables. Nearly half of the people in the survey ate no fruits and vegetables! A more recent survey by that same group revealed that not much has changed in the past few years. Even in the land of fruits and nuts (and vegetables) they don't eat their veggies.

The National Cancer Institute obtained more encouraging results when 32% of the people they surveyed claimed to be eating four servings a day of fruits and vegetables. I'm betting a big percentage of those people lied to the surveyors thinking the NCI would give them cancer if they didn't hear the kind of results they wanted.

Since people aren't likely to be easily persuaded to give up their current eating habits, why do so many experts continue to deny the health benefits of supplements? It's time the experts who worry so much about our pocketbooks and pee pee, face up to the fact that the cost of three to five servings of fruits and vegetables—depending on the location, the season and the produce chosen—is often more than the cost of a good multivitamin/multimineral supplement.

Pass the supplements

I'm sure the blame for the antisupplement sentiment can be attributed to Hippocrates who said, "Let food be thy medicine and medicine be thy food." Even though the great sage lived 400 years before the birth of Christ, many Ists still follow the dogma. Recently some experts were asked to list their choices of the healthiest foods. Not surprisingly, they all agreed that the best path to health is to "eat a varied and balanced diet." (And you thought sportscasters use annoying clichés.) Having said that, the food pros listed their top picks for choice chow.

Almonds were a big hit because they are supposedly rich in zinc, selenium, copper and potassium. They thought eight to ten nuts every other day would suffice but cautioned folks about eating too many because almonds are high in Calories. Thirty almonds contain about one metric thing of zinc. All multivitamin/multimineral supplements give you a daily dose of five to 15 metric things of zinc and no Calories. Supplements are also a far superior source of selenium and copper.

Blueberries were also a top choice due to their antiaging effects, their role in preventing cancer, delaying gray hair and wrinkled skin and improving memory and motor skills. A half cup two or three times a week was recommended with the stipulation that folks be sure to brush their teeth.

"What's with Poindexter lately? His teeth are turning blue."

"I asked him how he was feeling. He just smiled that cerulean smile and said 'berry good'."

Blueberries are among the most expensive berries and aren't available year round. A good antioxidant supplement costs pennies a day and is available 365 days a year.

Flaxseed and flaxseed oil were also high on the list because they contain fiber and some important unsaturated fatty acids. The Ists said to avoid flaxseed oil supplements because they are controversial. Aren't all supplements? They also said not to use large quantities. They'd rather have you eat fish.

The experts told us one or two cloves of garlic a day is good because it contains allicin, which is an antioxidant that helps lower cholesterol. If you're worried about vampires then keep some garlic hanging around and pull off some cloves as needed. Otherwise, inexpensive garlic supplements contain all the allicin you need and won't offend your friends' olfactory senses.

Olive oil was a top pick because it has one of the unsaturated fats we need and it lowers the bad cholesterol without affecting the good stuff. "Here, puppy. Aren't you a cute little fellow?" The Ists tell us to use olive oil sparingly because it's high in Calories. Yeah, it's fat.

The experts praised the benefits of salmon because it has unsaturated fatty acids that can reduce the risk of heart disease by lowering cholesterol. "Bad puppy. You shouldn't poop in Mommy's closet." Salmon is also good for the brain and nervous system. We're supposed to aim for three meals a week but we have to be very careful because salmon can have high concentrations of toxins—especially female salmon (salmonella). Omega-3 fatty acid supplements contain no toxins and accomplish the same things.

Sweet potatoes once or twice a week made the list because they're a good source of vitamin A and beta-carotene. So are multivitamin/ multimineral supplements and you can take them every day and not worry about tiring of the taste.

Tomatoes, the experts tell us, are a good source of vitamins A and C and they contain an antioxidant (lycopene) that protects against cancer and heart disease. We're supposed to eat a half cup every day or at least five days a week but we're not supposed to use ketchup because it contains sugar and salt. There's barely enough vitamin C in a cup of tomatoes to prevent scurvy and certainly not nearly enough to provide all the other antioxidant protection attributed to this important vitamin. I'm not convinced lycopene is any more effective than any of the other antioxidants that have been shown to prevent cancer and heart disease such as vitamins C and E, both of which are present in copious quantities in multivitamin/multimineral supplements.

As expected, the Ists put soy on their list but failed to supply any warnings. They apparently haven't been reading current literature.

Two or more servings per day of foods containing whole grains were recommended to prevent cancer and heart disease. Whole grains are certainly nutritious but even though they're not refined they don't provide the amounts of vitamins and minerals needed in our bodies to fight off disease.

As far as drinks are concerned, the experts said we should drink at least one cup of green tea each day to get a supply of antioxidants. For your information, all tea has similar benefits. Supplements also contain a good supply of antioxidants and you don't have to spend five minutes steeping to obtain maximum benefits.

The other drink suggested by the Ists was low-fat or skim milk (chocolate is acceptable) to obtain calcium and vitamin D. For those who can't or won't drink milk they mentioned kale and collard greens (which are a kind of kale, which is like cabbage), tofu, canned fish with soft bones or calcium-fortified juices and cereals. Nothing was said about the ease of taking a calcium citrate supplement.

Those Perturbing Pimps

Why, when there is abundant evidence at hand showing the benefits of supplements, do so many health professionals continue to ignore the facts? Surely it has nothing to do with a question of safety. Nutritional supplements have caused one recorded death, due to a massive overdose, in the last fifty years. Prescription drugs are responsible for approximately 125,000 deaths a year.

Is it because of the self proclaimed "experts" who sell vitamins and minerals to their friends and neighbors? I sympathize with the professionals who get rancors from entrepreneurial aspirants who profess to possess great knowledge of nutrition and nutrients as a result of purchasing a "kit" provided by a multi-level marketing organization. Toting their propaganda door to door, theses multi-level missionaries promise anybody who will listen everlasting health and wealth if they will join their team and buy their supplements. At huge rallies these would be J. P. Morgans listen to motivational speakers who urge them to get off their butts and get out there and sell, sell, sell. Some of the speakers tell them that our farmlands have been pillaged and raped while our food is processed and refined into undernutriented (now there's a word) masses of organic glob.

"Go ye unto the masses and save the flocks from the ravages of disease," and while you're at it sign up a few of the suckers so the company can reap more profit.

Is it the oleaginous chumps you see on late-night infomercials? Dressed in their tailor-made suits with dark hair oiled back, almost rubbing their hands with cupidity, they pimp "a new, state of the art vitamin/mineral supplement" containing vitamins and minerals you never even knew you needed. And, of course, their product is specially formulated for you. Thousands of people are being subjected to this crap, each with totally different nutrient needs, but the miscreants promise a special formulation for each one of us.

Or is it the journalist turned nutrition expert? After writing a book or two telling us how to eat and what supplements to take to enjoy everlasting health and happiness, these folks usually end up marketing their special brand of supplements. Without any testing of their "special formulation," these folks brazenly claim the greatest health benefits ever devised by God or man. Right on.

Again I sympathize with those who have spent years educating themselves about the body's needs and how to best fulfill those needs. Watching amateurs, in search of lucre, trying to perform a service that should be left to trained individuals causes bitterness. But this is America, a capitalistic society where everybody has a chance to attain wealth. Unfortunately, too many do it in the name of health.

I, like anyone who writes books, especially nutrition books, have the newest, best ever, guaranteed to work or your money back, cutting edge, state of the art solution. There's an old adage about attracting more flies with honey than vinegar (in this case the flies are folks). How 'bout all nutritional scientists and health professionals admitting to the fact supplements provide benefits? Sanction the sinners who haven't eaten all their fruits and vegetables but have at least tried to stay healthy with a vitamin pill. Follow this with suggestions (no dogma) to eat a variety of foods and take a good vitamin/mineral supplement every day. Rather than looking for ways to criminalize supplements, spend some time looking at the formulations hyped by the multi-levels, the infomercials and the journalists (experts who study journals) turned nutritionists (I can't believe I used that word). Do some price and product comparisons and publicize the results without bias or rancor.

Follow my suggestions and your problems are solved (or your money back). Professionals advocating and actually prescribing supplements would create a demand for high quality products. The gobbledygook touted by the slicks in the infomercials, the multi-level missionaries and the prose peddlers will have to pass muster or they'll soon be out of business. The American people would appreciate an end to the supplement debate.

On second thought, my scheme won't work until the professionals can agree on how much of each nutrient we need to obtain optimum health. Oh well, the best-laid plans.

One More Thing

Moments before I was going to push the button that would electronically whisk the text of this book to the publisher, an article appeared that begged comment. According to the report, physicians in a clinic located in the Southwest are recommending an untested supplement to their cardiac patients. Yes, you read correctly. Physicians with medical degrees from prestigious universities hanging on their walls, wearing their white jackets with their stethoscopes draped around their necks are going to sit in their offices and tell people there's no need to visit the pharmacy because they can call an 800 number and order a supplement to treat their heart disease.

The product hasn't undergone extensive clinical testing but that's okay because it's a proprietary formula, designed by doctors. This, of course, is supposed to make the uninformed think the supplement is oh so very special. And what makes it special? Nothing. The physicians who designed the formula read about studies conducted with omega-3 fatty acids, niacin, folic acid, a few other vitamins and some minerals. Nutrients that had positive results in clinical trials were put in the formula. The formula is referred to as an evidence-based nutraceutical, which means the product hasn't been tested clinically but its individual ingredients have.

The arrogance of these people! One of the principal objections advanced by physicians regarding supplements was the supposed lack of clinical tests. The docs just never bothered to read the journals that published the studies demonstrating the positive results obtained with supplements. Furthermore, for years Drs. Linus Pauling, Richard Passwater, Jeffrey Bland, Earl Mindell and a host of others examined the results of studies done with herbs, fish oils, vitamins and minerals and told people nutrients could be used to prevent and cure disease. They were scoffed at and labeled as quacks by many in the medical profession.

Why the change in attitude among physicians? Because entrepreneurs in the supplement industry have invited them to lunch, sent them samples and shipped them off to resorts for "educational" seminars. At these lunches and seminars the physicians are told that nutrition is a highly controversial subject and lay people need the sage advice of highly trained professionals. Never mind the fact the average physician has little training in nutrition. The company will supply all the training they need, at no cost to the professional. Nothing new here; pharmaceutical companies routinely and constantly employ the same tactics.

So now, physicians, apparently falling on hard times and recognizing the possibilities in an $18-billion-a-year industry, are designing and recommending supplements. Will this bring down the cost of drugs? Keep in mind, after Dr. Quackentalk makes the diagnosis, the good doctor will tell the patient about the heart disease and, smiling broadly, inform the poor soul she/he can make a choice as to treatment; either an obscenely high-priced drug of questionable efficacy or a much cheaper, untested nostrum.

Not all physicians, however, are jumping at the chance to become "experts" in nutrition by promoting and designing supplements. Physicians critical of their colleagues' "crossing over" are fearful that the number of medical doctors who condemn and admonish supplements might be diminishing rapidly. Worse, they fear, nutrition might actually become legitimized by the entry of MD's into the field.

The American Medical Association is whining about the ethical question of promoting health related products from the office. Isn't that rich? For years, doctors have diagnosed patients in their offices, prescribed an appropriate drug for treatment, sent them to the pharmacy to fill the prescription and then purchased stock in the company that manufactures the drugs they prescribe. This really is a wonderful country!

Ask the Expert

In this, the penultimate (look it up if you must) chapter, we're going to tap into the Internet to learn more about what nutrition experts do. The following is a collection of posted exchanges culled from websites operated by certified Ists.

Q: I've heard that cardiovascular exercise can prolong life. Is this true?

A: Your heart is only good for so many beats, and that's it, don't squander them away on exercise. Everything wears out eventually. Speeding up your heart will not make you live longer; that's like saying you can extend the life of your car by driving it faster. Do you want to live longer? Take a nap.

Q: Should I cut down on meat and eat more fruits and vegetables?

A: You must grasp logistical efficiencies. What does a cow eat? Hay and corn. And what are these? Vegetables. So a steak is nothing more than an efficient mechanism of delivering vegetables to your system. Need grain? Eat chicken. Beef is also a good source of field grass, a green leafy vegetable. And a pork chop can give you 100% of your recommended daily allowance of vegetable slop.

Q: Is beer or wine bad for me?

A: Look, it goes to the earlier point about fruits and vegetables. Beer is a liquid vegetable. So is vodka for that matter. Beer is made by feeding yeasty beasts barley and hops. After the yeasts are full of beer they pee it out and the brew master collects the vegetable-laden excrement in bottles and cans. Vodka is made from rotten potatoes, which are vegetables. Wine is made from grapes, which are fruits. Therefore wine is a fruit. Like wine, the fruit of the vine, gin is also a fruit. Gin is made from juniper berries, which are the fruit of the pine.

Q: How can I calculate my body to fat ratio?

A: Well, if you have a body, and you have body fat, your ratio is one to one. If you have two bodies, your ratio is two to one, etc.

Q: What are some of the advantages of participating in a regular exercise program?

A: Can't think of a single one, sorry. My philosophy is: No pain, good.

Q: Aren't fried foods bad for you?

A: People, you're not listening. Foods are fried these days in vegetable oil. In fact, they're permeated in it. How could getting more vegetables be bad for you?

Q: What's the secret to healthy eating?

A: Thicker gravy.

Q: Will sit-ups help prevent me from getting a little soft around the middle?

A: Definitely not! When you exercise a muscle, it gets bigger. You should only be doing sit-ups if you want a bigger stomach.

Q: I've heard chocolate is a vegetable. Is that true?

A: O.K. Just one more time with the veggies. Chocolate is derived from cocoa beans. Beans are vegetables. Sugar is derived from either sugar cane or sugar beets. Both are plants, which places them in the vegetable category. Thus, chocolate is a vegetable. To go one step further, chocolate candy bars also contain milk, which is dairy. So candy bars are a health food. Chocolate-covered raisins, cherries, orange slices and strawberries all count as fruit, so eat as many as you want. Chocolate has many preservatives. Preservatives make you look younger. If you get melted chocolate all over your hands, you're eating it too slowly.

Q: What's an infarction?

A: Please. There may be children accessing this site.

Q: We're leaving on a cruise soon. How can I control my weight?

A: Stay home unless you're willing to embark as a passenger and disembark as cargo.

Q: Any hints about remodeling my kitchen?

A: My next house will have no kitchen, just vending machines and a large trash can.

Q: What is your feeling about all these health fads?

A: Eat well, stay fit, die anyway.

Q: What's a balanced diet?

A: A cookie in each hand.

Q: Are there any advantages to bottled water?

A: I often wonder about those people who spend $2.00 apiece on those little bottles of Evian water. Try spelling Evian backwards.

Q: I do whatever my Rice Krispies tell me to, is that OK?

A: You! Out of the gene pool!

Q: I know salt and pepper are two of the seasons. What are some others?

A: Spring, Summer, Fall, Winter, parsley, sage, rosemary and thyme. Is it time for your medication or mine?

Q: If walking is so good for you, then why does my mailman look like Jabba the Hut?

A: He's obviously breaking the Calorie Commandment: Thou shall not weigh more than thy refrigerator.

Q: There is so much controversy about what causes heart attacks. What are your thoughts?

A: Heart attacks are God's revenge for eating Her animal friends.

Q: I've heard colloidal mineral supplements will protect against bio-terror attacks. Is that true?

A: The gene pool definitely needs more chlorine.

Q: I would like to build up the muscles in my arms and shoulders. Any tips?

A: I'll tell you my boyfriend's, the big hunk, secret for building arm and shoulder muscles. Start by standing with a five-pound potato sack in each hand. Next extend your arms straight out to your sides and hold them there as long as you can. Do this three days in a row then move up to ten-pound potato sacks. Do this five days in a row then move to 50-pound sacks ten days in a row. Finally, lift a 100-pound potato sack in each hand and hold your arms straight out. Do this until you can hold your arms out for more than a full minute. This might sound like real work, but the results are worth it. After the workout with 100 pounders, start putting a few potatoes in the sacks, but don't overdo it at this higher level.

Finally

This is the chapter you've been waiting for with baited breath. I spent hours trying to find the origin of this term but was unsuccessful. I was going to lie and tell you the exact origin was unknown but it was thought to have come from Minnesota or maybe Louisiana or Georgia and it had something to do with men who fished a lot. That was until I learned the phrase is "bated breath," which means you've been holding your breath right up until now. Please exhale.

The time has come for me to give you my recommendations for a healthy daily intake of vitamins and minerals and compare my recommendations with the RDAs (not to be confused with the U.S. RDAs) and RDIs which were once the U.S. RDAs but aren't now because they are the DMVs whose job is to issue license plates and driver's licenses.

To devise my recommendations, which I call the EATS (Eat All This Stuff), I borrowed numbers liberally from the National Research Council, the FDA and various authors (no journalists or physicians turned nutritionists though).

As you see, the table has a lot of footnotes. That's because scientific tables always have a lot of footnotes at the bottom. Sometimes there are more footnotes than numbers in the table. Often there are so many footnotes one needs a magnifying glass to read them. So you won't need a special lens, I've asked the publisher to place my footnotes on a separate page in normal typeset. You're welcome.

A Table (but no chairs)[1]

Nutrient	RDA[2]	RDI[3]	EATS[4]	Comment[5]
Vitamin A	1300 RE[6]	5000 IU[7]	5001 IU	Footnote 8
Vitamin D	200 IU	400 IU	401 IU	Footnote 9
Vitamin E	12 IU	30 IU	400 IU	Footnote 10
Vitamin K	80 mcg[11]	80 mcg	81 mcg	Footnote 12
Vitamin C	95 mg[13]	60 mg	500 mg	Footnote 14
Thiamin	1.4 mg	15 mg	20 mg	Footnote 15
Riboflavin	1.6 mg	1.7 mg	20 mg	Footnote 15
Niacin	18 mg	20 mg	100 mg	Footnote 15
Vitamin B_6	2 mg	2 mg	20 mg	Footnote 15
Folate	400 mcg	400 mcg	800 mcg	Footnote 15
Vitamin B_{12}	2.8 mcg	6 mcg	30 mcg	Footnote 15
Biotin	35 mcg	300 mcg	301 mcg	Footnote 15
Pantothenate	7 mg	10 mg	50 mg	Footnote 15
Calcium	1000 mg	1000 mg	1200 mg	Footnote 16
Magnesium	420 mg	400 mg	421 mg	Footnote 17
Phosphorous	700 mg	1000 mg	1001 mg	Footnote 17
Chloride	750 mg	3400 mg	3400 mg	Footnote 18
Chromium	50-200 mcg	120 mcg	400 mcg	Footnote 19
Copper	3 mg	2 mg	3 mg	Footnote 18
Iodine	200 mcg	150 mcg	201 mcg	Footnote 18
Iron	30 mg	18 mg	15 mg	Footnote 20
Manganese	5 mg	2 mg	6 mg	Footnote 18
Molybdenum	250 mcg	75 mcg	150 mcg	Footnote 18
Selenium	75 mcg	70 mcg	200 mcg	Footnote 21
Zinc	19 mg	15 mg	5 mg	Footnote 22
Choline	550 mg		550 mg	Footnote 18
Sodium	500 mg		800 mg	Footnote 18
Potassium	2000 mg		3200 mg	Footnote 18
Fluoride	4 mg			
Boron			3 mg	Footnote 20
Germanium			?	Footnote 20

[1] Here we go with the footnotes already.
[2] RDA is the acronym for Recommended Daily Allowance.
[3] RDI is the acronym for Recommended Daily Intake.
[4] EATS is the acronym for Eat All This Stuff.
[5] This is a table with lots of footnotes.
[6] RE is the acronym for retinol equivalents. I have a Ph.D. in nutritional biochemistry and can't understand them.
[7] IU is the acronym for international units. Let's leave it at that.
[8] Did I mention that vitamin A is a hormone?
[9] Vitamin D is a steroid hormone but it's legal.
[10] Vitamin E, the stud-muffin vitamin. Take the highest level.
[11] A mcg is a microgram, which is one millionth of a gram, which is .000000036 ounces, which is pretty small.
[12] Could've been named the Dam vitamin.
[13] A mg is an English made sports car. It's also 1/1000 of a gram which is .000036 ounces.
[14] The RDA and RDI for vitamin C are O.K. if you're an abandoned sailor.
[15] The RDA and RDI for the B vitamins might have suited the cave dwellers but not modern she's and he's.
[16] This is not just an udder nutrient.
[17] Also used in fireworks.
[18] No comment.
[19] 400 mcg hooked onto picolinate or it's worthless.
[20] More research is needed.
[21] Selenium is a potent antioxidant. Go for the big one.
[22] If it's zinc picolinate, 5mg is all you need!

Section Three:

GLOSSARY AND APPENDIX

Stuff Ists Never Learned in School

Glossary

Abdicate: To give up all hope of ever having a flat stomach.
Adipocytes: Lipid larders.
Artery: The study of painting.
Balderdash: A rapidly receding hairline.
Benign: What you be after you be eight.
Bacteria: Back door to cafeteria.
Barium: What doctors do when patients die.
Carcinoma: A valley in California, noted for its smog.
Catscan: Searching for Kitty.
Cauterize: Made eye contact with her.
Cesarean Section: A neighborhood in Rome.
Coffee: A person who is coughed upon.
Colic: A sheep dog.
Coma: A punctuation mark.
Congenital: Friendly.
D&C: Where Washington is.
Diet: Special food for those who are thick and tired of it.
Dilate: To live long.
Enema: Not a friend.
Esplanade: To attempt an explanation while drunk.
Fester: Quicker than someone else.
Fibula: A small lie.
Flabbergasted: To be appalled over how much weight you have gained.
Flatulence: The emergency vehicle that picks you up after you are run over by a steamroller.
Flummery: Oatmeal or flour boiled with water until thick.
Gargoyle: An olive-flavored mouthwash.
Genital: Not Jewish.
G.I.Series: World Series of military baseball.
Glossary: A list of terms in a special field, subject or area, with accompanying daffynitions.

Hangnail: What you hang your coat on.
Impotence: Nature's way of saying, "No hard feelings."
Labor Pain: Getting hurt at work.
Lymph: To walk with a lisp.
Medical Staff: A doctor's cane.
Morbid: A higher offer than I bid.
Nitrates: Cheaper than day rates.
Node: I knew it.
Outpatient: A person who has fainted.
Pap Smear: A fatherhood test.
Pelvis: Second cousin to Elvis.
Pokemon: A Jamaican proctologist.
Post Operative: A letter carrier and part-time surgeon.
Rectitude: The formal, dignified demeanor assumed by a proctologist immediately before he examines you.
Recovery Room: Place to do upholstery.
Rectum: He damn near killed him.
Rheumatic: Thinking of love.
Secretion: Hiding something.
Seizure: Roman emperor.
Tablet: A small table.
Terminal Illness: Getting sick at the airport.
Testicle: A humorous question on an exam.
Tumor: More than one.
Urine: Opposite of you're out.
Varicose: Near by/close by.
Vein: Conceited.
Vegetarian: A person who will eat nothing that has a mother. (If vegetarians eat only vegetables do humanitarians eat…?)
Willy-nilly: Impotent

Appendix 1

Every credible book about nutrition has an appendix, and a liver and a hepatic vein and a reticuloendothelial system. The appendix in a human is essentially worthless. Similarly, the appendix in a book contains worthless information that was difficult or impossible to insert in the main body. Also, some of the material in an appendix is redundant, which makes these sections redundant sections.

Fact: The Japanese eat very little fat and suffer fewer heart attacks than the British or Americans.

Fact: The French eat a lot of fat and also suffer fewer heart attacks than the British or Americans.

Conclusion: Eat what you like. It's speaking English that kills you.

We should really be more careful about where we stick our ists. If a nutritionist studies nutrition does a capitalist study capitals? Is a motorist a mechanic who studies motors? Does a sexist study...well you get the idea.

I'm in shape. Round is a shape.

Practice safe eating habits. Always use condiments.

It just occurred to me that the reason most scientific names were taken from Greek is lawyers had the Latin (*pro bono*, *caveat emptor*, *et cetera*, etc.) and the scientists didn't want to get involved in litigation.

O.K., what's the speed of dark?

Nutrition science is an oxymoron but my all time favorite is Microsoft Works.

On the other hand, you have different fingers.

If you yelled for eight years, seven months and six days you would have produced enough sound energy to heat one cup of coffee. (Hardly seems worth it.)

The human heart creates enough pressure to squirt blood 30 feet. (Whoa!)

A pig's orgasm lasts 30 minutes. (In my next life, I want to be a pig.)

A cockroach will live nine days without its head before it starves to death. (Creepy. I'm still not over the pig.)

Banging your head against a wall uses 150 calories an hour. (Do not try this at home…maybe at work.)

The male praying mantis cannot copulate while its head is attached to its body. The female initiates sex by ripping the male's head off. ("Honey, I'm home. What the…?!?")

The flea can jump 350 times its body length. It's like a human jumping the length of a football field. (30 minutes…can you imagine???)

The catfish has over 27,000 taste buds. (What could be so tasty on the bottom of a pond?)

Some lions mate over 50 times a day. (I still want to be a pig in my next life—quality over quantity.)

Butterflies taste with their feet. (Something I always wanted to know.)

The strongest muscle in the body is the tongue. (Hmmmmmm...)

Right-handed people live, on average, nine years longer than left-handed people do. (If you're ambidextrous, do you split the difference?)

Elephants are the only animal that cannot jump. (OK, so that would be a good thing...)

A cat's urine glows under a black light. (I wonder who was paid to figure that out?)

A pessimist's blood type is always B-negative.

Dijon vu - the same mustard as before.

Does the name Pavlov ring a bell?

A successful diet is the triumph of mind over platter.

When you dream in color, it's a pigment of your imagination.

Reading while sunbathing makes you well-red.

Support bacteria. They're the only culture some people have.

A clear conscience is usually the sign of a bad memory.

Change is inevitable, except from vending machines.

Health nuts are going to feel stupid someday, lying in hospitals dying of nothing.

During hours swimming at a municipal pool, you will ingest 0.4 gallon of urine.

In an average day, your hands will have come into indirect contact with 15 penises (touching door handles, etc.).

An average person's yearly fast food intake will contain 12 pubic hairs.

In a year you will have swallowed 14 insects—while you slept!

Annually you will shake hands with 11 women who have recently masturbated and failed to wash their hands.

Annually you will shake hands with six men who have recently masturbated and failed to wash their hands.

In a lifetime 22 workmen will have examined the contents of your dirty linen basket.

At an average wedding reception you have a 1/100 chance of getting a cold sore from one of the guests.

Daily you will breathe in one quart of other peoples' anal gases.

Sharing a bag of crisps with a friend gives you a 10% chance of ingesting a small amount of their feces.

Appendix 2
Quotes

"My doctor told me to stop having intimate dinners for four. Unless there are three other people."
-Orson Welles

"No diet will remove all the fat from your body because the brain is entirely fat. Without a brain, you might look good, but all you could do is run for public office."
-George Bernard Shaw

"Food is an important part of a balanced diet."
-Fran Lebowitz

"We are living in a world today where lemonade is made from artificial flavors and furniture polish is made from real lemons."
-Alfred E. Newman

"I was a vegetarian until I started leaning toward the sunlight."
-Rita Rudner

"You can tell a lot about a fellow's character by his way of eating jellybeans."
-Ronald Reagan

"There is no sincerer love than the love of food."
-George Bernard Shaw

"What is food to one man is bitter poison to others."
-Lucretius

“If we could give every individual the right amount of nourishment and exercise, not too little and not too much, we would have found the safest way to health.”

-Hippocrates c. 460 - 377 B.C.

Appendix 3
Nutri rhymes

It's a very odd thing—
As odd as can be—
That whatever Miss T. eats
Turns into Miss T.

Walter de la Mare, English poet and novelist.

Jack Spratt could eat no fat,
His wife could eat no lean,
And so betwixt them both,
They licked the platter clean.

John Clarke a.k.a. "John the Baptist" from the 17th century, about 1639.

Printed in the United States
17738LVS00002B/91-153